PENGUIN BOOKS
STOP WEIGHTING

RAMYA SUBRAMANIAN is a well-known anchor, actor and also a fitness icon based in Chennai, Tamil Nadu.

She is the founder of Stay Fit With Ramya, a YouTube Channel and an online platform that now provides holistic health, fitness and nutrition programs for Indian women living all over the world.

After winning gold in the district- and state-level powerlifting championships, Ramya is so much more than a media celebrity today.

Ramya got her CPD credits and completed her certification course at IIN, New York, last year and is now a certified Integrative Health Coach.

With Love,
Ramya

06/12/2022

ADVANCE PRAISE FOR THE BOOK

'*Stop Weighting* by Ramya is a book which succinctly portrays her tryst with destiny filled with drama, intrigue, and inspiration. This multi-talented woman has taken a multi-directional approach to life, which augments her cerebral pursuit. Right from being an anchor to an actor, her approach speaks of hard work. In the process she has found time to write a book which is her fitness diary filled with emotions, strategies, and experience. Kudos to Ramya for bringing her efforts to light through this lens; it is going to be a pathbreaker.'

—**Basu Shankar, former strength and conditioning coach for the Indian cricket team**

'Ramya's first book *Stop Weighting* is a delight to read. Reading it was like going to a therapy session with a talented psychiatrist who themselves had fought depression but had come out successfully in the other end. It is relatable, making the whole experience authentic. I enjoyed the exercises at the end of every chapter immensely.'

—**Suhasini Manirathnam, actress**

STOP
WEIGHTING

a *guidebook* for
a fitter, healthier you

RAMYA
SUBRAMANIAN

PENGUIN BOOKS

An imprint of Penguin Random House

PENGUIN BOOKS

USA | Canada | UK | Ireland | Australia
New Zealand | India | South Africa | China

Penguin Books is part of the Penguin Random House group of companies
whose addresses can be found at global.penguinrandomhouse.com

Published by Penguin Random House India Pvt. Ltd
4th Floor, Capital Tower 1, MG Road,
Gurugram 122 002, Haryana, India

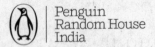

First published in Penguin Books by Penguin Random House India 2022

Copyright © Ramya Subramanian 2022

10 9 8 7 6 5 4 3 2 1

The views and opinions expressed in this book are the author's own and the
facts are as reported by him which have been verified to the extent possible,
and the publishers are not in any way liable for the same.

ISBN 9780143455035

Typeset in Bembo Std by Manipal Technologies Limited, Manipal
Printed at Thomson Press India Ltd, New Delhi

www.penguin.co.in

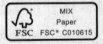

*To my creator
Who blessed me to seek out my darkest fears
and to write about them here with courage*

Contents

Part II

Laying the Groundwork for Your Fitness Journey

Part III

Fitness Myths and Methods

Part IV
Your Guidebook to Nutrition

Part V
Mind Your Mind

Disclaimer

The author is not a health care practitioner or a nutritionist. All information provided is purely for informational and educational purposes. The information is not intended to treat, cure or prevent any disease/disorder and will not provenly make the reader healthier/gain or lose weight or muscle mass. All the information provided in this book is solely based on the author's personal experiences and opinions and should not be interpreted as an attempt to offer a medical opinion. The author and the publisher of this book are not responsible for any adverse reactions, effects or consequences resulting from the use of any recipes or suggestions herein or procedures undertaken hereafter. If readers have questions about food, diet, nutrition, natural remedies or holistic health, they are requested to conduct their own research and consult with their health care practitioners. Readers who are pregnant, nursing, have a medical condition or are taking any medications are requested to consult their health care practitioners before making any changes to their diet or supplement regimen.

Trigger Warning

Some readers may find discussions in the text on depression, anxiety, eating disorders, sizeism or fat shaming as triggers.

Introduction

Dear Reader,

Hello! How are you doing?

First and foremost, I'd like to take a moment to thank you for buying this book. Of the millions of books out there, you've chosen this one. That means a lot to me.

Over the years, I've received a lot of love from people around me and have felt the need to give back in a small but, hopefully significant way. That is how this book came into being. To every woman and man out there who has come and spoken to me or has written to me about their helplessness in the health and wellness aspect of their lives, this book is written because of you and for you!

I initially had my qualms about writing this book, but I feel a strong sense of responsibility to motivate, uplift and share my experiences and to address a lot of the misinformation circulating out there with regard to health and fitness.

Now, let's get down to business.

This isn't one of your magic 'weight loss mantra' books that guarantees you will lose 10 kilograms in 10 days. Nor will it put you on crash diets that will make you 'shrink instantly' or get a flat belly.

This book is entirely about my story—situations I have faced both as part of my life and fitness journey since the days of my childhood up until now. It is about how I handled challenges and what I learnt from them, the hard way. Integrated into that are guidelines I believe will help in managing your weight and mental health and ensuring your well-being.[1] I've also shared a sample workout, a generic nutrition plan and plenty of recipes to help you kick-start a holistic approach towards good health, balanced nutrition and happiness.[2]

Finally, I have shared some glimpses from my life and the challenges I face working in the media. I have written honestly and candidly, and to the best of my ability.

In a certain way, this book took me down memory lane and opened up an episode from my life that was locked up and left untouched for a long time until now.

Now, let me tell you my *kutti* (little) story . . . but first a few things:

---

[1] These guidelines may not necessarily produce results when used by others.
[2] The workout, diet programme and recipes have been curated as a general good practice that worked for me, without keeping the individual readers' dietary/medical/nutritional needs and requirements in mind. Readers must consult their dieticians/nutritionist/doctors before incorporating these changes into their lives. Also, any product recommendations are based on my own experience and are not paid endorsements.

How to Use This Book

Writing this book has been an eye-opener for me. Thanks to my parents and the sacrifices they've made, I've lived a secure and steady life for the most part. But I've also had my fair share of moments when life has relentlessly thrown difficulties at me. So, dear readers, I hope you will consider this book to be much more than just a 'timepass' read. This book is a sincere, direct and heart-to heart conversation between you and me based on my life experiences and my research.

This story is mine, but I'd like you to focus on what *you* can take away from the experiences I've shared. It would be best to read this book at a stretch without skipping chapters, to underline key points and to jot down summaries of your own thoughts and takeaways. After you've read each chapter, I urge you to take a few minutes to reflect on what you've just read. See how you can implement some of these things in your own life. Hoping that what took me 10 years to understand and rectify may take you only 10 months!

In this book I've included tables with supplementary information on health, fitness and well-being along with exercises that encourage you to diligently and openly write down your thoughts and feelings. I strongly believe in the power of writing—it helps solidify your goals and take them more seriously. Even if this slows down your reading to one chapter a day, that's okay. Do it! Do not skip, for your own sake! WRITE IT DOWN!

Finally, while the information I've shared here comes from experience and research, it is my duty to caution you to never venture into anything blindly. Seek guidance from experts and professionals where necessary to ensure you're on the right path to achieving your goals.

We're about to begin a beautiful journey together—one that's special and exciting and goes straight from my heart to yours. If this book can make even a little bit of difference and make you feel happier, stronger and more fulfilled, I'll consider my mission accomplished!

Happy reading!

Yours,
Ramya

Part I

The Highs and Lows of My Fitness Journey

#1

My Beautiful Reader

I am a 100 per cent bona fide original and that is the biggest high for me today!

But that wasn't the case always. An entire series of events unfolded to make me the woman that I am today. I used to be insecure, shy and constantly anxious about the way I looked. There was a time when, if I had to wear something tight and uncomfortable during a shoot (because I didn't have the guts to refuse back then), I would have nightmares about it afterwards. I'd obsess about how my love handles would be on display for the world to see, or how I'd be ridiculed and body-shamed by people who watched my show. I would cry myself to sleep with these worries whirling around in my head; when the show aired, I'd refuse to watch it because I hated the way I looked. Clearly, my self-love score was in the negative at the time!

People around me, including some who didn't know me at all, took it upon themselves to point out my flaws. They would tell me how I 'looked dull' on a day (when I'd actually be in the best of spirits); how I had a 'terrible zit' on my face; how 'good girls don't get into media'; how I 'looked better in person than on TV' (hold on, should I take that as a compliment?). I have been pointed at and commented on—how my head is big for my body, how I am disproportionately built, and once someone even told me how I'd get more offers if I got a nose job!

The first time you hear such things, it hurts. The second time, it makes you cry. The third time, you fall apart. But after the fourth time, you simply become numb to all the noise, and that is exactly what happened to me. After an incredibly long time, I've finally come to realize that the mantra to looking good is 60 per cent confidence, 20 per cent style and 20 per cent the smile and attitude you carry.

The confidence and strength that people sometimes say they admire in the 'new' me is a result of treating myself the way I feel I deserve to be treated. I want to look good for myself and ensure I lead a happy life with no regrets. I want to prioritize my health because I love myself (and this is me today, after succumbing to a lot of self-destructive criticism in the past, which you will read about in the later chapters). That is why I exercise every day and try to eat as healthily as I can. Yet, there are those rare days on which I am still affected by the nasty comments and brutal language of others, for I'm still human at the end of the day. I have found that the best way for me to handle such negativity is by choosing not to read, listen or watch content that bothers me.

When I feel I deserve to indulge myself for my discipline and dedication to my workout and nutrition regimen, I go buy that dress I've had my eye on for a while or indulge in that decadent chocolate fudge that everyone's been raving about. Basically, I plan my indulgences and gift them to myself time to time!

Embracing a healthy lifestyle, being the best judge for your own body's needs and finding a balance in life are key. I know that my body acts a certain way when I get hungry; I recognize the urge to eat out of hunger (rather than anxiety or boredom) by the little signals that my stomach sends me every three to four hours like clockwork. When that happens, I immediately make a healthier choice now to eat something filling and nutritious than go on a binge eating food that does not make me feel satiated. The healthier option could be food that I would have meal-prepped or stocked up on earlier or a delivery from an eatery but one where I consciously choose a smarter option from the menu (thank God every restaurant has a health hub list these days) without any hesitation. I know now that this is the way my body functions. I have noticed how other people prefer a long gap of five hours or more between their meals just so that they can have a big meal at one go. No hard and fast rules here about the right or the wrong way. They have become accustomed to a certain system that is different from mine. You need to find a way that is sustainable and practically workable for you. What I can vouch for is that the tricks of stocking up on nutritious food in advance and not let tempting foods lie around the kitchen or refrigerator help. Try these tricks out and you will agree too!

I remember the time when as a seventeen-year-old I walked onto the set of my show holding my mother's hand and got stopped by the cameraman. He pulled me aside and asked me if I had partied hard the previous night. I was shocked at his suggestion, but when I dismissed it he made fun of me. He even called me a liar and went on to say that he could sense how much booze I had had just by looking at my face and belly! In reality, I had spent the whole of the previous night preparing for my semester exams and the consequence was the puffiness in my face. But to this man, my face and belly fat were evidence of having indulged in alcohol. This and many other such incidents truly shattered me as a teenager and it took a very long time for me to throw off the burden of such nasty comments and memories. What all this leads me to say is that it is important to start owning one's weaknesses. Very often, these are the things that distinguish us from others and make us strikingly original—our body fat, our acne and skin issues, how we stand, how we walk, how we pose—everything! JUST OWN IT. Every single person perceives things differently and it is not our job to explain ourselves to a world that decides to dissect every bit of information about us and then comments on it.

It's the same story with women and make-up. Each of us has a certain type of face and skin tone, and so a 'one-size-fits-all' make-up routine simply doesn't exist. The very thought of the days back when I'd get caked with make-up for my show still has me breaking out in a sweat! I now understand that my face looks better with little or no make-up. I like it when the unevenness, the marks and the pigmentation of my skin are visible. All of it is part of who I am, so I choose to own it rather than camouflage it. Here, I must include a note on actor Sai Pallavi: When she first appeared as Malar in the Malayalam film *Premam* owning her beauty with absolutely no make-up on her, it was extremely refreshing to watch someone so relatable. Being her authentic self has become her identity and

I respect her tremendously for being a natural beauty in the world of cosmetic attractiveness! Here's a great example that the natural and original definitely go a long way.

And so, my dear reader, I encourage you to embrace your natural beauty. Do not be hard on yourself no matter what anybody thinks or says. You don't have to explain or prove your worth to anyone if you are aware of it yourself.

Exercise

List five traits that make you a complete original:

1. _____

2. _____

3. _____

4. _____

5. _____

2

'You Are Fat'

Nobody likes hearing the words, 'You are fat.'

I was 15 when those words were hurled at me for the first time. But before we go into that story, a little background.

I was a geek in school. Oily hair, thick spectacles—you'd never have given me a second look. My friends called me 'Thayir Sadam' (curd rice), 'Soapu Moonji' (soap face) and 'Paal Dabba' (milk tin). I was one of those frontbenchers who'd scream out the answers to all of the teacher's questions, and that would annoy my classmates to no end!

Back home, I would eat non-stop, without any control. I was a 'growing child', you see, so up until a certain point, I was allowed to eat without restriction. In retrospect, the overeating might have been an early sign of my anxiety or of an impending eating disorder.

Read my school textbooks and eat a sandwich or samosa, with French fries on the side.

Watch TV and eat ghee dosa, poori, instant noodles, chilli cheese toast or pizza.

Play video games and eat—actually, be fed by my mom—curd rice, rasam rice or paruppu rice with potato roast.

This was my routine and menu, every single day.

Other than my Bharatanatyam classes, I didn't engage in any physical activity. Actually, for the amount I ate, the fact that I could hold my body together and move during my dance classes was a huge feat. My dance teacher would constantly tell me to lose weight so that I could at least fit into my dance sari. (I needed to drape the pallu of the sari around my hips and tuck it to the side; but with my broad waistline, I was never able to wrap the pallu around myself fully!)

When I'd start crying about this, people around me (except for my teacher, that is) would console me. They assured me that I looked cute that way, and they called me 'Amul Baby' and told me to just ignore everything and stay just the way I was. The moral of the story: Never fall into these traps. They do you more harm than good. Just as body shaming is bad, I think celebrating someone who is growing to be unhealthy is not good either.

As a result of living this big fat life throughout my school days and adolescent years, I became overweight, and it was obvious that I was headed down the wrong road. It wasn't until my dad pointed it out to me and took a strong position on it that I finally started to become aware of the facts myself.

However, initially I didn't respond well even to his views on what I was doing to myself. I used to feel deeply hurt when my dad told me off for spending hours sitting in front of the TV just like my brother (but he was physically active and I wasn't!). Every time my dad saw me eating junk food, he insisted that I exercised. I was a very sensitive child and felt crushed when I was prevented from enjoying the relationship

I had with food. I did not have friends and neither did I have the drive to learn a craft; all that mattered to me was eating junk food. The comfort that food brought me, no person could. I was so annoyed with dad for policing my food habits that I foolishly decided to take revenge on him by eating more and becoming even more of a couch potato. I mean, what an idiot I was, right! That silly teenage ego!

I continued to eat in this way and gained weight uncontrollably till my weight hit around 65 kg. And then, something happened . . . something I will never forget. I had just finished my 12th standard board exams and my mom took me out shopping to celebrate. We were in the teenagers' section in a shop. I really liked a top at this store and asked for my size to try it on. The attendant gave me a look, then went into the storeroom and took out the top in XL size for me to try on. When I couldn't fit into it, she told me (somewhat kindly, to soften the blow) that that was the largest size they had in the store. If I wanted to find clothes I could fit into, then I'd better look elsewhere.

That was a real slap in the face. Even today, I see it as one of my biggest embarrassments—so much so that every time I visit an apparel store, I pause for a moment at the kids' section. I understand that stores are divided into different sections according to age and gender for the sake of convenience. But isn't it important for them to also be mindful of including a range of sizes to cater to men and women of all shapes and sizes? Who decided that a certain person of a certain age should be able to 'fit into' clothing of a certain size? I request brands to be more sensitive and inclusive of clothing for both men and women, for those who are skinny as well as those who are large; especially in the case of kids, because incidents like the one I just described can take a heavy toll on a child's fragile self-esteem, the way it did for me.

I came home and cried and cried. Until then, I had never taken my weight issues too seriously. When my friends made fun of me and even when my dad pointed it out, I brushed the criticism off, assuming they were all just jealous that I was happy and enjoyed my food. But with that one shopping experience, the message hit home brutally, because it came from a store attendant who was an outsider and who did not know me and did not care if she ruined my happiness with her remark. Also, she made her comment in the dressing room area, where other moms and kids were looking at me in surprise, as if they were perplexed about how someone my age could be so 'overgrown'. Up until then I was the spoilt and pampered teenager who always got all she wanted thanks to her hardworking and extremely loving parents. But now, even if externally nothing stopped me from getting that top I really liked, my own body became the reason I didn't want to buy it!

That was the starting point of me feeling insecure with my body. I became deeply depressed for a long time after that. I stopped wearing ready-made clothes altogether. I switched to salwar suits so that I could fully cover up, and would specifically instruct the tailor to make them 'loose' and 'droopy' so that I'd look thin in them!

I retreated into a shell. I stopped going out and meeting people and stopped talking to my family at home. I felt like the whole world had turned against me. Looking back now, I feel that maybe I needed to go through all that before I could eventually find my own way out. Perhaps I should have spoken to my dad about it and asked him for help. Maybe I should have started becoming more active.

I can trace my every response to body image issues back to the time when my identity became that of a 'fat' person, because that is what I felt people viewed me as. Me being overweight should not have been anybody's problem except mine, but when everyone feels entitled to comment on someone else's body, an extreme reaction such as mine—only a child at that time—is only to be expected.

When we are kids we are conditioned to identify food as a reward for doing well in examinations and sports or for being obedient to elders. We also get treats on our birthdays and so on. These stay etched in our memories for the rest of our lives and this is why our brains come to associate food as an incentive. As adults, we are led by this conditioning to often fall into the trap of emotional eating—using food for comfort, treating food as medicine for depression and anxiety, and relying on food to lift us out of loneliness and boredom.

We can change the way we think of rewards. How about taking the child out to a play area with recreational activities or spending more time with them doing something fun like coaching them on how to play badminton, teaching them how to cycle, swimming together, taking them on a jog to the park with you or even taking them out on a holiday or to a nearby zoo or museum? Apart from helping us strengthen the bond we have with the little ones at home, time spent together in this way also helps the child look up to us. By being the best examples of how to take care of ourselves we can show our children how to do the same. It is when we become lazy and don't get involved with them, choosing to make them happy with decadent desserts and the latest PlayStation, that the problem starts.

Now I am not saying that we should restrict children and not allow them to eat what they want. But I guess what I am trying to explain is that we should help children develop a balanced mindset and value self-care. As parents, we are responsible for our children up to a point, and how we raise them and the foundation of habits that we help them build are what set our children on the path of growing on their own in future.

Being fat is not the problem.[1] The problem is letting them remain fat because they are just kids, or reacting to it in an offensive and insensitive way that would hurt them by leaving deep scars.

Five Tricks That Can Be Practised with Young Children to Stop Overeating

1. Chewing the food and eating slowly.
2. Preferring full meals to small, low-calorie nibbles (because you keep getting hungry when you graze and also tend to consume more calories mindlessly).
3. Including a balanced proportion of fruits, vegetables and lean proteins in each meal.
4. Eating mindfully, in a distraction-free way (and that also means no gadgets or eating outside the dining area).
5. Limiting indulgences and outside food (both ordering in and going outside for a meal) to one meal in a week.

---

[1] From an obesity point of view, caused by an unhealthy lifestyle and overeating. This does not refer to weight gain due to medical issues such as thyroid, PCOD and other health issues which children may have less control over.

Exercise

No one really forgets the first time they got teased for their body being a certain way. Write your own experience of the time you were first taunted about how you looked.

_____

_____

_____

_____

_____

3

I Want to Be a Supermodel

Welcome to phase two of my immaturity.

Now, where were we? Ah, yes. So, I continued to get oversized clothes tailored for myself, which made me look at least 10 years older. I also started to become unsocial. I refused to attend friends' birthday parties, weddings or family functions, and stayed in my room whenever we had visitors over—I was afraid that people would comment on my looks and tell me to lose weight, which would depress me even more. This insecurity also started to affect the way I interacted with my parents, and I would keep conversations with them to a minimum.

One other thing happened: I started feeling ashamed of eating in front of others. As a result, I ate little when my parents were around and went through the fridge or the kitchen late in the nights when no one was there to help myself to leftover food. In other words, I started enjoying eating alone and in secret where nobody watched what and how much I ate.

Although my parents were concerned about my strange behaviour, they attributed this change to that typical 'teenage phase' which I seemed to be going through and hoped that I'd outgrow it at some point. And so, things continued like this for a few months. The more I got teased and mocked about my appearance, the more shut-in, insecure and miserable I became. The worst part was that I didn't have the guidance I needed to change things. So, my insecurities were bottled inside me and kept transforming from one issue to another.

But when I least expected it, things took a turn. After around six months, one day, I fell ill with severe food poisoning. I was throwing up and feeling nauseated no matter what I ate or drank. Being very naive then, I concluded that God had finally decided that I'd had enough food for my entire life and was sending me a sign to stop eating. But when I didn't eat anything for three consecutive days and still didn't get better, I had to accept that this definitely wasn't the case. It was then that I tested positive for jaundice.

Hello and welcome to phase jaundice! This phase was, in some ways, a turning point. It changed a lot of things about the way I ate, and consequently, the way I felt about myself.

The next two months were excruciating. I survived on orange juice, sugarcane juice and bland idlis day in and day out to flush out the infection. In the process, my weight dropped drastically by 10 kg to 55 kg. What happened next gave me the courage to actively pursue weight loss.

Friends and relatives began to take notice of this radical change in my size. Suddenly, I looked 'great' and 'amazing' to them. (The irony was that I was still recovering from jaundice and felt weak and fatigued all the time!) They kept asking me how I'd lost so much weight, and begged me to share my secret with them. The neighbourhood boys, who earlier barely knew I existed, were now giving me second glances whenever I walked by. One boy, whom I had always addressed as 'Anna' (meaning brother), came up to me one day and told me to stop calling him so! This was a confusing phase for me; on the one hand, I looked pale and ill, had no appetite, felt like shit, was throwing up all the time and had absolutely no energy; and yet on the other hand, all that mattered to the people who saw me was how thin I looked and how much weight I had lost!

I found myself in the spotlight for the very first time in my life. Regardless of how shallow the attention I received from people was, I was busy trying to live up to it because I had never felt appreciated for my looks before, nor had I been noticed by members of the opposite sex until then.

This is when my fixation on trying to get as thin as possible started, because in my mind

Being thin = Being liked + Getting attention.

I started exploring ways of appearing thin using outfits, and becoming thin by starving myself and over exercising. People from the profession I chose to be part of also kept telling me that it was always good to lose a few kilos no matter how thin one was (because the camera adds extra weight too!). (Of course, this was unhealthy and I don't advise it.)

In fact, it took me a long, long time to get past the false correlation between being thin and being liked as there was no body positivity or body neutral movement back then.

But if you think after this I got things right and started eating well and exercising regularly, you are mistaken, dear reader. You see, I had for the very first time tasted the rush of receiving attention from other people and I was not going to give it up. From being an 'Amul baby' with a problem of overeating, I swung to the other extreme of becoming desperate to lose more and more weight to fulfil my need for validation.

It became an unhealthy obsession.

How Did I Start My Fitness Journey?

1. It began with an alarm that rang inside me. It felt like my body was telling me that it had tolerated enough of my abuse but hadn't given up on me yet.
2. I cut back one by one on my unhealthy eating habits: overeating, starving, eating out of stress/anxiety/boredom, etc.
3. I followed a few good Instagram handles on nutrition and fitness to keep myself motivated and get the guidance I needed.
4. Every morning, I planned my day's healthy eating (to keep myself away from junk food) as well as my exercise (walking, going up and down the stairs 10–15 times) and tried to stick to it.
5. I sought help from a professional nutritionist and a personal trainer.

Exercise

Have you ever made it a habit of setting up a regular time in your calendar and engaging in a physical activity at that time almost every day in the form of a sport, walking, workout, etc.? If your answer is yes, note down the pros and cons of how you felt when you started, and what made you stop (if you did stop):

PROS	CONS
For example, felt energetic and refreshed	For example, had no motivation for the next day's session
_____	_____
_____	_____

4 4

4

As Long as I Can Be Thin

As a health coach now, I get to talk to and understand the mindset of my clients who come from different demographics and psychographics.[1] I find that no matter how much we emphasize and create awareness on having the right mindset towards our bodies, the younger generation is still heavily invested in the mantra, 'It is important to lose weight to look good'.

When I see youngsters desperate to lose weight, I feel responsible to help them understand that this isn't a good sign and it is not the correct way in which weight loss should be perceived. And to help them understand this, I often use the stories from my own life—the foolish things that I have done and their consequences.

After I recovered from jaundice, my goal was very simple: I had to find ways to become the slimmest version of myself.

---

[1] I am a Certified Integrative Health Coach, with a degree from Institute for Integrative Nutrition, New York. You can find more about my health coaching on Instagram at my handle @stayfitwithramya.

I was determined to fit into smaller-sized clothing and I went all out trying every 'diet plan' that there was.

This was around the time when the Internet was opening up whole new worlds for me, and it quickly became my window to a host of diets: the then-popular 7-Day GM Diet, the Cabbage Soup Diet and the Lemon Juice Detox Diet, to name just a few. I diligently took printouts of all of these and started following them.

I also consulted a few dieticians and some of them endorsed the most outrageous diet plans. I remember this one dietician who saw me at a friend's birthday party and smiled. When I smiled back at her, she asked me how old I was. Even before I could answer her, she said I looked 26 to her (I was 18, a full 8 years younger!). There went another night of good sleep. And not just that. While I was finally working on my confidence and self-esteem, this 'dietician's' remark pushed me back to a place where I didn't want to return. I hid my tears but I'm sure she saw my eyes getting moist. She held my hands and said I looked hairy and bloated; she said she had asked me my age out of the concern that I had PCOS (polycystic ovary syndrome)—which, by the way, I never even knew about until then. She asked me to visit her clinic the next day and gave me her business card. So, I went with my mother.

At her clinic, she took out a big box with no label on it. She filled it up with an assortment of pills, explaining that if I took them twice a day, they would help me lose 5 kg and that it was the cure for my PCOS. Only later did I learn two important things from my gynaecologist: Firstly, I didn't have PCOS at all, and secondly, PCOS cannot be reversed; only its effects can be reduced by maintaining a good lifestyle involving exercise and balanced nutrition. But back then, given my frame of mind, I fell for the dietician's recommendations blindly without even asking her what pills she had just given me and why the box was not even labelled! I'm thankful that this didn't do me much harm (or so I think), but I shudder to think about the risks I had taken being completely unaware.

Another dietician suggested that mere deep breathing would help me lose all the excess body fat. I could eat whatever I wanted to, but just had to take a few deep breaths before and after each meal. There went Rs 10,000 straight out of my pocket. (Err, it was my mom's purse back then!)

I also recollect the time when I was a newcomer in front of the camera. I'd get super anxious about my outfit before a shoot. Wearing tight-fitting, unflattering outfits got on my nerves and my discomfort was evident to all; but I'd simply go along with it. Later, after the show was telecast, I was body shamed by viewers—they'd comment on how the outfit made me look—and I would go deep into my shell. That's when the co-anchor of the show suggested the then-popular 'lime juice diet' to me. As the name suggests, you simply sip on as much lime juice as you want to, all day long. And that is all you get to drink for the whole day. My co-anchor told me that it helped her stomach flatten briefly and was some kind of a skin detox too and helped the skin glow. Of course, I tried the diet. A day before and on the day of every shoot for about six months, I was sipping away on lemonade, not realizing that the sugar in it was spiking up the insulin level in my blood. As a result of this diet, I felt low on energy all through the day. Even something as simple as walking up to the shoot location a few times would tire me out. I constantly wanted to pee, but had to control it, and this didn't do my bladder any good! I would feel claustrophobic, and the smallest of things would annoy me. Imagine a 20-year-old going through all of this!

The days following the lime juice diet were very rewarding—I would drop almost a kilo. But, the 'fruits' of my labour were short-lived. After my first solid meal, my weight would immediately shoot up again! For all that effort and pain . . . sigh! This cycle didn't stop until the producer of my TV show noticed I was doing this on every shoot. He called me aside and gave me a piece of his mind. He warned me that I was setting myself up for diabetes at a young age.

From all this, you must be able to tell how much I had craved and surrendered to the idea of thinness, which was exploited by people who lacked insight and were unprofessional and unethical. In retrospect, I can't help but feel that they preyed on my vulnerability, like many astrologers do when a distraught family comes to them for 'redemption' from their misery.

The results of following these crash diets were obvious. I would lose weight substantially in the first few days, but there were numerous side effects that plagued me:

- I constantly felt tired and too exhausted to do anything.
- I experienced anxiety, mood swings and frustration.
- My skin felt dry and flaky; hair fall increased day by day; my nails were chipped and broke easily; and the skin around my nails peeled away.
- I developed severe digestive issues. I fluctuated between days of diarrhoea and constipation, and constantly looked bloated.

- My menstrual cycle became irregular with very poor blood flow.

Although the diets worked while I was on them, the minute I stopped, I gained double the weight I'd lost in just a couple of days. I also observed that the more frequently I was on these diets, the more difficult it became to lose the weight. My body had started becoming resistant to and intolerant of all the experiments I was putting it through. My metabolism went for a complete toss.

I felt that problems were swallowing me up again. Despite all the torture I was putting myself through, the same people who'd complimented me on my weight loss just a month earlier would tell me that I'd put on weight again. I felt helpless and had no idea how to handle it all. As a result, I often obsessed about the little details: Was it the dress I wore? Was it the last meal I had? To make matters worse, the diets affected my moods so terribly that I couldn't continue them beyond a week or two. Nobody could understand what I was going through and I was too embarrassed to discuss things with anyone.

Clearly, the diets and crash diets weren't helping. Any sensible person would have stopped there. But the desperate Ramya in me didn't give up.

5

Work (Out) Your Ass Off

Our brains are wired in a way that we dislike losing things; but the one thing that goes against this principle is our desire to LOSE WEIGHT! This desire was very strong in me too and I wasn't ready to give it up!

After about two years of pursuing every conceivable crash diet (more on these in the next chapter)—all of which failed in the long run—I finally realized that they weren't working for me. I came to this conclusion when I accepted that diets were hard to sustain.

Among the difficulties I faced were practical issues. I did not want to eat the same food over and over. Neither could I eat at exactly the same time every day like the diets recommended. Given my anxiety and constant mood changes (which were side effects of the super strict diets), not compromising on the portion sizes was a huge struggle. Worse still, accessing some of the food items that these predominantly Western diets advocated—such as kale, celery, zucchini, blueberries— required great effort as they are not easily available in India!

These diets were becoming expensive and difficult to follow. Also, I would easily get bored of a diet and look for the next one that had worked for someone, hoping it would help me too!

My next plan of action was to lose flab by going all out on EXERCISE mode.

This was the time when all of our heartthrob heroes had their best six-pack bodies on display—the *Ghajini* and *Sethu* era. During interviews, the actors would talk about how they'd built their bodies through extreme workouts.[1] Being starry-eyed and stupid, I was completely swept off my feet by all of this. I couldn't afford a professional trainer, of course, but I made up my mind to achieve a perfect body all on my own, without guidance from anyone.

To inspire and motivate myself, I plastered the walls of my room with posters of beach-body babes (the ones you'd normally find in boys' rooms). I would wake up to them, stare at them for hours on end, and fantasize about having the same chiselled body, wearing those sexy swimsuits and glamorous clothes.

I took the obvious next step—joining the gym and going crazy with workouts! Pursuing something with passion and determination is a good thing. But being hyper obsessed is never good. My obsession with working out was unnatural and was a sort of addiction. And any kind of addiction is a bad thing.

---

[1] See   https://www.indiaglitz.com/suriya%C3%82%C2%92s-special-training-for-ghajini-hollywood-news-13187;   https://caravanmagazine.in/vantage/vikram-transforms-characters-i.

From the day I stepped into the gym, people took notice of this irresistible urge in me when it came to working out in a certain way and following a specific regime. Everyone wanted to be out of my way and would leave in a hurry the moment they saw me enter. Some would even call up the trainers to check my gym schedules for the day, so that they could choose an alternative time!

A few unwritten rules quickly fell into place for me when working out.

1. I requested trainers to switch off the AC as soon as I walked in. I wanted to sweat every second that I was in the gym and I felt that I could evaluate how successful my workout was based on how much I sweated during the session. I was under the illusion that the more I sweated, the more effective the workout was.

What my younger self from 10 years ago didn't understand was that a good workout had nothing to do with a pounding heart rate or pouring sweat; these only create a sense in some of us that we have achieved something important.[2] It is more the endorphin release and feeling of accomplishment that I look out for in a sweaty session today.

2. I had the music in the gym changed from the usual international playlist to a 'Biriyani' list of back-to-back local *Marana Mass Kuthu* (high-octane energetic commercial film songs) tracks. I'm a true Tamilian that way . . . In fact, I still prefer a local commercial song to the *Rocky* soundtrack when

---

[2] See https://timesofindia.indiatimes.com/readersblog/rachit-sharma-fitness-on-does-sweating-burn-calories/does-sweating-burn-calories-39228/.

I want to feel charged up and lift heavy weights. You'd know if you follow me on Instagram!

3. Until I finished my session, everyone else would stay away from the equipment (for their own good!). I would thump heavily with my flat feet on the treadmill and the deafening sound would literally chase everyone away. Back then, I didn't know how to jog or sprint, and I guess the trainers were too reluctant to knock some sense into me.

I would take endless amounts of time on the treadmill, EFX and cycling machines, so that no one could use them until I finished my session. And as there were only a few such machines in gyms back in those days, this made matters worse for others. (If you are one of these people reading my book now, I'm sorry—please forgive my insensitivity and entitlement!)

How long I'd run on a particular day would depend on my mood. If I had felt okay in my clothes the previous day, I would target burning 500 calories, which took approximately 45–50 minutes of jogging at 10 km/h. But if I'd eaten a large meal or someone had commented that I looked like I had gained weight, all that rage would come out and I'd run at an insane speed of 12 km/h for as long as my body would allow. (By the end of the book you will find out how I handle such comments about my weight nowadays.)

Just my cardio workout took anywhere between one to two hours. After that, I pushed myself to do about 200–300 abdominal crunches, 200 oblique crunches with the stick and 200 leg raises for about 30 minutes. I thought that the more crunches you did, the more quickly the fat in the abdominal areas melted away.

Well, what can I say? That's how fixated I was back then to become the slimmest version of myself.

People tried educating me and talking to me about the injuries I'd sustain by working out like this, but seeing me pay no heed, they eventually gave up. To this day, my friend actor Samantha, who watched me go through all of this, reminds me how crazy I used to be, running like a mad woman on the treadmill!

I am incredibly blessed and grateful that despite torturing my body with excessive workouts and crazy diets, nothing went severely wrong. I'm pretty sure that it was good genetics and my young age which allowed my body to handle all that abuse I heaped on it. I thank God for my parents' prayers, which helped me get through this body-damaging phase without any major repercussions.

(PS: I was recently told that there are quite a few people in my gym who, following my lead, now ask for the ACs to be switched off when working out. My coach has been thanking me for saving the gym's electricity bill. Well, instead of just thanking me, maybe you could consider reducing my membership fee too? Just saying!)

The Truth about Fat Loss

STOP THIS ✗	START THIS ✓
Extreme crash diets and starving	Balanced calorie-deficit diets
Fat burner supplements	Sleep and reduced stress
Cardio in excess	Weight training and a little cardio

6

When I Lost It, I Didn't Lose It!

That's right. The crash diets, the long and intense workout sessions at the gym, the growing desperation and the ever-present sense of insecurity were becoming unbearable and I was getting more and more frustrated.

To lose weight I did everything possible . . . and I mean EVERYTHING!

Apart from my infamous gym sessions, I would go for long walks in the mornings with a group of neighbourhood uncles and aunties. They would religiously start at 5 every morning, but it was too hard for me to wake up at that hour. I would still drag myself out of bed, even if I hadn't slept well the previous night. This meant that even if I found the walk hard and I was groggy and tired the rest of the day, but I just could not give up.

Then someone told me about Zumba, a fun dance form of cardio, and I dived in immediately. As much as I enjoyed some fun dancing around, adding this to my already punishing schedule of early morning walking and sleep deprivation didn't help me perform to my optimum. Next, I met a friend who had lost a lot of weight doing aerobics, so off I ran in that direction! All of this was just me adding several routines of cardio to my day. My muscle damage was obvious in how weak I felt when I had to stand and host my TV shows/events and shoot for hours.

After trying out everything, I decided to calm my inner senses and as a coach suggested, I started yoga for inner peace and also practised breathing which would contribute to 'faster' weight loss. I quit after two days—'it's way too slow' and 'I don't have the patience for this' were my excuses that time! The real reason, however, was that I lacked balance and flexibility; my body felt so stiff as a result of all the cardio sessions that yoga, being the opposite of all that, was something that I couldn't nail in one go! My body and mind were making so much noise that letting go and surrendering to calm my senses seemed impossible back then. It made me feel like a loser and I ran away from yoga instead of trying to work on it to improve myself.

* * *

I've already told you about some of the crazy diets that I resorted to, but there are a few that deserve special mention for the sheer level of harm they cause to one's health. One of them was called the 'Blood Type Diet'. As its name suggests, in this your diet is decided based on your blood type and it was quite popular at the time I attempted it. The idea was to choose foods compatible to one's blood group as each belongs to a certain evolution age period.

So, I said to myself, 'Let's do this!' Unfortunately, my blood group, O positive, is the ancestral blood group in humans and belonged to the hunters, which meant that the only foods I was supposed to eat were meat, fish, poultry and a few specific fruits and vegetables. But I was a vegetarian from birth. So, needless to say, this diet didn't make sense to me. I did try for 12 days, surviving on raw vegetables and apples like hunter vegetarians (even dairy was not allowed in the diet!) and concluded that I would rather die being myself than mimic the popular eating strategy of hunters!

Another one I tried was the Military Diet. Of all the diets I'd tried, this one was my favourite! The Military Diet allowed me to have ice cream as part of my meals for the first three days, and for the next four days, I could choose from a whole range of options. The diet allows small portions of food that we all enjoy and indulge in as treats, but keeps a check on our overall calorie intake, and that's how we lose weight. The problem with this diet though was that like many other diets, the weight would climb back up the moment we went off it. Since it includes sugar, dairy, processed foods, I'm not sure how healthy it can be for someone who has food sensitivities and intolerances. Also, it didn't emphasize on the quality of food; all that mattered was to eat fewer calories even if the meals were unbalanced, lacked vitamins, nutrients and minerals, and would give rise to deficiencies.[1]

---

[1] See https://www.verywellfit.com/the-3-day-military-diet-review-3495299#:~:text=Cons%20of%20the%20Three%2DDay%20Military%20Diet&text=May%20not%20provide%20enough%20nutrients,considered%20a%20healthy%20diet%20plan.

I wouldn't recommend any of these diets. There simply isn't anything sustainable or sensible about them. Today, having understood the science behind fat loss, I realize how an extremely simple straightforward process that requires some self-discipline has been made to appear complex by multinational companies that endorse crash diets for their own gains. We as consumers (sadly, mostly women) continue to fall for these ploys, because of the pressure to look a certain way.

When the chemistry between my entire body and its fuel (food) fell out of gear, worrying signs started showing up internally and at times externally. My hair was thinning, I had constant gut problems, my nails were brittle and broke often, my skin felt dry at all times, I had dark circles and lines under my eyes because of the lack of sleep. A 19-year-old should not be showing any of these symptoms, but this was me! I succeeded in briefly camouflaging these signs with make-up for my TV shoots, but people who saw me without make-up, including my college classmates, constantly asked me why my face looked puffy, why this, why that. I was on the verge of a breakdown trying to come up with answers while coping with the relentless scrutiny.

Here's a list of all the misconceptions and insecurities I had as a teenager and for most of my twenties.

I thought eating after 8 p.m. would make me fat.

I also thought skipping breakfast would make me fat.

After I started intermittent fasting, I used to think eating breakfast would make me fat.

At one point, I thought eating fat would make me thin and eating carbs would make me fat.

I even thought protein would make me fat, destroy my kidneys and bulk me up.

I thought all artificial sweeteners were poison.

I thought calories didn't matter.

Later, I thought calories were all that mattered.

I thought doing abdominal exercises was the way to getting six-pack abs.

I thought protein shakes were steroids.

I thought I knew everything there was to know about fitness.

I fell for each and every myth, fad, diet, workout, pill, potion and powder.

I fell for all of them.

And if you're reading this, you probably have too.

Which is kinda ok because we all make mistakes.

We all mess up, and above all, we all fall for nonsense.

But as long as you're trying, regardless of the challenges, you'll win.

That's what helped me rise above all of this. You must be shocked reading all that I had put my body through. But it was important for me to learn all of this to work anew on myself. So, I don't regret any of it and I don't want you to beat yourself up if you too can relate to me now.

7

The 'Aha' Moment

I'm now taking you back to the day when I was called for an audition for a television commercial. That was the day everything changed about the way I treated my body until then. This must have been at least 7 years ago. When the script was given to me, I was taken aback to find that the role was that of a mother of three, the eldest child being 12 years old. He was right there, and when he looked at me, I tried to imagine what it would look like if he called the then 24-year-old me 'Amma' in a commercial that more than 6 million people would see. I just couldn't complete the audition. I told them that I was not feeling well and ran back home.

I looked into the mirror and cried . . . Why was this happening to me?

Why did the casting manager choose me for the role of a woman who had a 12-year-old child when my own age was 24? Did I look like a woman who was in her thirties to him? It goes without saying that the career of an actor or model depends a lot on their looks. The problem in this case was not that I had to play the role of a mother of three kids. Maybe if the same offer came to me now, I would accept it. No, the issue was that I looked older than what I really was. For the fragile person I was back then, it broke my self-confidence.

I did not like what I saw in the mirror. No matter how closely I watched what I ate or how intensely I worked out, I felt I was no closer to the face and body that I dreamt of. I had tried everything I could think of and yet nothing had really changed. I thought that I perhaps needed to quit my job to start respecting myself better and not let people break my self-esteem.

I cried and cried until my eyes were red and I couldn't cry anymore. I decided to postpone the idea of chasing my body goals, because I had reached a point where it was too much to handle and was completely losing myself. I decided to accept myself for what I was and not chase after what I didn't have. I had no more energy and excitement for it anymore.

And there was one thought that kept getting reinforced: I was the problem. I felt that while other people were able to follow the diets and get results, I didn't get my desired result because I was either not doing it right or I lacked will-power and commitment.

I wanted to press a button that could reboot everything for me to start over, only this time with some better decisions. 'One day at a time, Ramya'—this was my mantra (and it still is!).

I cried myself to sleep. I woke up the next day determined to make a new beginning. My first thought was to mend my health which was not in a good place. Several things were going wrong: I was eating too little, not sleeping well, overdoing my training, losing my hair, getting dark circles, and all the while my weight was fluctuating.

I felt I could start with a good sensible trainer to guide me. Until then, everything I had tried was my own random efforts based on what I had read, heard or seen, which is a mistake a lot of people like me still do. I had never gone to an expert for guidance. Do not underestimate the knowledge a good coach brings with them—from helping me understand my body correctly and knowing what works and doesn't work for me, making me accountable and keeping me on track, to customizing a programme based on my body's condition and my goals. The whole mess started to untangle itself when I took coaching from the experts. In the end, this was the wisest decision I made, and it marked the real beginning in my fitness and health journey that has brought me to where I am today.

It is important to be in the right hands and do a bit of research. Follow the experts or ask those who have trained under them before signing up with them. I did that too. I discussed my problems with my training coach and nutritionist, and the advice I got in return was very simple: If my body was not responding to all my efforts, then my failure was possibly linked to some kind of food allergies, slow metabolism, misguided training, stress and lack of sleep. When I started, I was asked to train only three times a week so that I could get a good eight hours of sleep, and to stop eating all gluten foods as there was a lot of wheat in my diet. That is all I did. I switched from rotis and parathas to millets and rice, and I rested more and relaxed, trusting the process. In about a week's time, my stomach started 'going in', my gut and tummy felt much lighter and my energy levels were great. This is what worked for me, based on my body type, metabolism and allergies.

Next, I was trained on conditioning exercises and stretches, and how to warm up before every session, something that I used to totally ignore earlier. Back then, I would simply walk onto the treadmill and start jogging without warming up or stretching. I didn't take time to cool down afterwards either. But this time, I started with workouts based on 'High Intensity Interval Training' or HIIT. I am sure you are familiar with burpees, bear crawls, kettlebell swings, snatches, etc. now, but back when I started, all of it was quite new. It was exciting to learn, apply and progress from the small weights to the next bigger one.

And yet, although I was losing fat rapidly, I couldn't see any definition in my muscles or even much increase in strength after the first few weeks. The reason was that my body did not get the essential protein requirements to recover and build muscles. I was a vegetarian who didn't even like eggs and getting the required quantity of protein every day through broccoli, paneer, soy, dal, tofu, legumes and lentils was impossible. On top of it, they made me feel heavy and gassy. Getting access to them every single day during shoots and remote locations was also a challenge. I had to resort to eggs and whey protein.[1]

Initially, I had my apprehensions about protein supplements just like most of you. Due to the very nature of our upbringing, we have been trained to be wary of ready-made off-the-shelf

---

[1] I am not endorsing that vegetarians have to turn to egg; they can have other supplements as well.

items and instead rely on traditional home-made or farm products. Moreover, protein supplements have had their fair share of controversy; some professionals insist we consume them while others don't. But since it was a trial period for me, I went ahead and bought whey protein and started on eggs. I was already eating four to five portions of vegetables, protein-rich foods and at least three litres of water, to which was added a scoop of protein powder in water and four egg whites in the afternoon. It became my new routine.

Now, when I woke up, I would look at myself every day, liking what I saw in the mirror and noting the change in my clothes' sizes too. I wanted to improve and see how much the protein intake could contribute.

Honestly, within 14 days of starting to have a scoop of protein powder after my workout and introducing eggs into my diet, I could feel a huge change in the way I was lifting weights, as well as in my hunger and satiety levels. The protein was a blessing for me; I was stronger in my workout sessions, I had a newfound energy that helped me stay positive and active, I was less hungry and I stopped craving for and binging on sweets. There has been no looking back at my belief in meeting with adequate protein intake ever since.

Having said this, I must ask you to never do something just because it worked for someone else. Don't go and get just about any protein powder immediately because I said so. Of course, there's no harm in trying it out, and if you see the results as I did, I am happy for you. But at the end of the day, remember that we are individuals and each of us are biologically unique in a way that only we can relate to ourselves. This is a fact I will keep reiterating at various junctures in this book.

For instance, I am fine with having a shot of black coffee when I wake up on an empty stomach. But some of my clients have a problem with acidity and I don't recommend it to them.

Similarly, whey protein has suited me just fine, but for some of you, it may cause acne problems or make you feel bloated. In that case, you can choose a vegan alternative (more on protein powders later in this book).

There are even those who claim that working out while you're fasting makes burning that stubborn fat easier. However, I won't recommend this arbitrarily to anyone, as my friends have told me they feel giddy in the mornings when they work out with me in the gym without having eaten anything.

I can't stress enough to you the importance of the right information and guidance. But just remember, don't consume anything you don't believe in, as that kind of approach won't do any good to your body. When you start out on something, be it a nutrition plan, an exercise regime or even a coach you approached, remember to start with a positive mindset and have faith in it.

8

Being a Unicorn

For nearly a decade, I had tortured myself with all sorts of nonsense, when the solution had been clear and simple all along.

Thank God I had the epiphany that the problem wasn't me but rather that I was trying to fit myself into an arbitrary universal diet and workout designed by people who don't know me, my lifestyle, my ethnicity, my metabolism or anything at all about me! When I found fault with myself and beat myself up about it, the problem turned back onto me. I was just blaming and shaming myself instead of trying to address the root cause for my self-sabotage.

When I realized this, I finally had my breakthrough and started seeing the results I wanted.

We all do this, right? Trying to force ourselves into a circle but not realizing that perhaps you are a square, your mom is a rectangle and I an oval!

If you're in this state now, my friend, you have my sympathies. It is hard for us to see the worth inside us on our own, and that is why having an expert showing us our worth from the outside is incredibly valuable. I realized that fitting myself into what was working for my friend, sister, mother or a celebrity I found on the Internet was not the solution.

The only way to a real and lasting change is a plan customized that is suited to me and my surroundings. And to learn that lesson, I had to put my body through so much!

In fact, I didn't even know the difference between exercise (workout) and training. Do you know the difference between these two terms?

Working out or exercising is anything that we do to move our body. It can be in any form: walking, swimming, sprinting, yoga, Zumba, aerobics, working out in the gym on my own or dancing! All the random things I was attempting earlier and shifting from one to another were different forms of exercises.

On the other hand, training is movement done with a specific purpose in mind.

For example, an athlete trains because their workouts are created for a certain reason. It can be to increase endurance, to improve their agility in the field or increase strength, to be able to add muscle to withstand long hours of playing, etc.

Any activity we do for fun, to get some movement into our routine and balance our otherwise sedentary lifestyle, is a workout. But in order to achieve a certain body goal, we need a training plan. Until I had a specific training plan that was aligned with my goal of losing fat and followed a balance calorie-deficit eating plan based on that training that was tailored to my height, weight, lifestyle needs, etc., I couldn't achieve the result I so badly wanted. No matter what I did and how much I strived, it just didn't work.

So, depending on what your unique goal is—fat loss, building strength, gaining muscle or even a maintenance plan to move to immediately after your fat loss—your eating and workout plan should be structured accordingly.

For instance, is your goal a mind–body connection aimed towards improving your flexibility? Then yoga is most likely the best plan for you.

Is your goal building strength and muscle? Then I would suggest weight training for you.

The question you need to ask yourself is whether what you are doing now is structured to create the results you want.

There is nothing wrong with workout programmes and there are a lot of inherent benefits in moving your body too. So, if that's where you are at and you just want to move your body every day, great! Choose what you love and enjoy and go with that.

But if you want your body to adapt in a certain way towards a specific result or a goal, then you need a guided training programme.

And it doesn't stop with a structured training plan alone.

Have you noticed that your eating habits—the way you eat, what and how much you eat—change from time to time? That's because even the preferences and needs of our nutrition evolve with age. I have noticed my own taste keeps changing. As a child I adored savouries and chips, salty and oily food but disliked chocolates and anything sweet completely. But now, sweets and desserts are my indulgences and I don't enjoy savouries like I used to.

Depending on your allergies, food preferences, location, BMI, ethnicity, gender, height, weight, etc., you need to understand your food choices and build a balanced eating plan.

The sooner you realize this the better. I do understand that money can be a concern and not everyone can afford a trainer, a gym, a dietician and a health coach. But when it comes to your health, I don't want to risk giving you any other suggestion that may turn out to be wrong. From what you've read so far, you know that I tried a lot of things that went wrong and made me waste my hard-earned money. Going to an expert was the only thing that straightened everything out for me in the end.

Moreover, if you are a beginner and have never received any training guidance, do not blindly follow workout videos on YouTube just because they are free. Most of my clients come to me with a history of injuries, muscle pulls, damaged knees and back, and we have to get them into rehabilitation for weeks or months to set them right!

This is why when I post a video of my regimes on YouTube, I weigh the consequences carefully and add my cautionary disclaimer in it repeatedly.[1]

Moving forward, you would do well to save up for your health regime. Thanks to the pandemic, we have become more attuned to paying attention to ourselves, and nothing should come in the way of us being healthy. When you plan out your monthly expenses, start adding two columns for WANTS and NEEDS. For a month, simply keep adding all your purchases under each of these two headings. Your necessity is a NEED, and what you spend for pleasure is optional and becomes a WANT. They can be your food, the cookies and chocolates you indulge in, the vacations you go on, the clothes, watches,

---

[1] See https://youtu.be/5tpRhVWI3b8.

bags and everything that you buy. You will soon understand how much money you can save to invest on a good coach for your health.

I'd like you to think about this carefully. Even if you can't spend much on your health currently, I'd still want you to start saving 10 per cent of your monthly income, considering the damage it will eventually spare your mind and body. Save at least that much until you can invest on a good coach someday sometime.

* * *

So many of us fall into the lie that the harder something is, the better it works. The more miserable we feel, the more our fat loss regime is working. That, my dear friend, is a losing strategy. That is why when life gets in the way, we find it difficult to sustain putting our body through that hardship. That is why we give up and lose all the progress we have made until then. If we are miserable, we will fail quickly too.

I want you to be successful in everything that you do and achieve every little goal that you've ever set. But to do this in a sustainable way, you need to enjoy what you do and not give up what makes you happy. When you start to like the way you work out and the way you eat, you will stick to your plan far longer, and then, imagine the results you will get! My plan worked for me only when I accepted it as a part of my life and not a favour that I was doing for my body.

On the first day of enrolment, my clients often have the mindset of giving up everything they love—sugar, snacks, pizzas, fries, all of it—due to their desperation to lose fat. I know it the minute they say, 'I'll do anything, give up anything you tell me to!' That sentence is a red flag for me.

You need not give up everything! You just need to have a plan on what is non-negotiable for you—the things that make you happy and that you are not willing to give up in pursuit of your goal. Can you work out for two hours every day for six days of the week for the rest of your life to lose weight? Or do you want to do it smoothly, taking gaps in between and being able to enjoy and have time to spend on other parts of your life as well? Will you be able to commit to 16 hours of intermittent fasting (IF) all your life? When we identify all those non-negotiables and integrate them into a plan completely designed for you, the plan works absolutely effectively.

However, if you most definitely cannot get an expert to help you at the moment, the best option is to stick to the basics and keep your goals small and simple to make progress.

Start slow. Use the guidelines provided in the 'Workbook' section of this book. Make slight changes to your existing patterns of eating and exercise, and observe the changes to your body and correct accordingly. Once you start seeing results, you can build from there and then seek help from an expert when you feel ready.

For example, if you eat junk food every day and have never worked out, your goal should not be to get six-pack abs, but to lose two to three kilograms in a month's time.

To achieve this goal, do simple things. Cut out junk food for a week first, and including more vegetables in your diet from the second week. Add 30 minutes of walking every day from the third week, and keep increasing your step count and hitting your targets. Join a challenge community group, and so on.

Tips to Start on Your Own

- Take a long brisk outdoor walk every day for an hour to include movement in your routine.
- Eat more of real foods and less of processed ones.
- Include lots of vegetables, fruits, proteins with moderate carbs and fats in your diet. Get in more of this and you will automatically crowd out the junk.
- Add a regime of deep breathing with long exhalations for at least five minutes a day.
- Sleep for eight hours.
- Drink plenty of water.

So far, all that you read is a gist of my errors since teenage years, my misguided attempts when I became desperate to fix my body aesthetically. You just read what happened when I disrespected my body and abused it.

Now, enough of that, let us begin with what to do to avoid that from happening.

Part II

Laying the Groundwork for
Your Fitness Journey

9

Owning How You Look

The first step towards fat loss is to understand why you want it to be gone. What is your goal? Why do you want to lose weight (or even gain weight, if that is what you wish to do)?

If someone had asked me this question a decade ago, my answer would have been:

- To be able to wear any outfit given to me and look stunning in it, without any flab popping out while I'm in the spotlight.
- To feel validated by my audiences, friends and family.
- To impress everyone.
- To have a tiny waist and have the Barbie doll body proportions (32-28-36).

I know that I realized pretty late in life that these can't and shouldn't be the reasons for wanting to be fit. A few other reasons for losing weight that I've heard from my clients are:

- Their daughter has a pretty face, but they think that she also needs a pretty body to find an appropriate life partner.
- They think of themselves as a loser in the workplace. People make fun of them, and the only way they think they can get back at them would be to have a good body.
- Their partner finds them to be ugly and so asks them to lose weight.
- Their friends make fun of them because of their body.
- They think that being thin is the most 'happening' thing.

I can go on and on, but it makes me upset to list these reasons. One of the most challenging aspects of our lives, especially for women, is embracing our bodies in all their shapes, sizes and colours. I feel that this conditioning to be ashamed of our bodies begins at school, with the behaviour of the people around us ingraining these problems in us. It is hard to move past these experiences because they are inculcated since childhood.

Growing up, I never felt content with the way I looked and always felt that there were certain standards of beauty that I had to meet as a girl. (This problem is not restricted to girls, but girls do tend to bear a disproportionate burden of adhering to accepted standards of beauty.)

First, several societal expectations are thrust onto young girls by our cultures—for example, the idea that we need to sit a certain way, tie our hair in a certain form, wear a certain kind of attire and not be too loud and so on.

Once you reach adolescence, a new set of expectations is imposed. There is a greater focus on physicality: you cannot be too plump nor too thin as that would presumably drive away potential grooms (and many times rejections start with the groom's folks who are part of the selection process); instead, you need to look a certain way in preparation for a partner who will desire and 'accept' you. I have an anecdote to share about this exact issue. The mother of a friend would tell her to skip dinner every day and only drink a tall glass of apple–beetroot–carrot (ABC) juice to maintain her physique. From the eleventh grade onwards, her mother would ask her to take steps to get fairer, suggesting that that would help her look her best while seeking her future life partner!

The pressure to trim and shape your eyebrows and shave your body hair starts to build up soon after this. I remember the time in high school when my close friends would ask me to shave my arms and legs, constantly commenting on how hairy I looked. I knew that they did not have any ill intentions as one does not know any better at that age. To make matters worse, my mother would never let me groom myself or go to the salon until I had almost completed my first year in college. So, this became an embarrassing problem to deal with that had no real solutions at the time.

Most of us live through adolescence in confusion, not knowing which side to lean on (the protective parents vs friends) in making our decisions, don't we?

Right after puberty, when I realized my hips were growing wider and my breasts were getting bigger, the changes to my body felt weird as it was not something I had been prepared for or warned about. This, on top of the prohibition of grooming, made things worse as I could sense that other kids were making fun of me and calling me unacceptable names. Straightening my hair, sporting the latest hairstyles and painting my nails were the next criteria to impress and attract the attention of the boys around me. At school, there were already these cliques in the class that you could not be a part of unless you looked 'cool' enough or measured up to a certain standard in the boys' eyes. All of this was an additional pressure for me to look a certain way just to fit in with the other children at school. It wasn't fair, but this is how these expectations at school become a burden while growing up.

Meanwhile, at home, parents tell children to minimize their distractions and ask them to stop thinking of the way they look and instead focus on obtaining good grades. Even when we get to the age at which we are allowed to make our own beauty choices, we don't receive proper guidance from our families. This is because these topics are not usually openly discussed with family members in our culture. For example, my mother used to recommend applying turmeric on my face whenever I asked her to help me with the problem of upper lip hair. Doing that just yellowed my face, which led to more ridicule from the other kids. I know our mothers do their best with what they know. They probably did not even get any guidance from their own mothers.

What do we do then?

If I could go back in time, I would not change anything about my experiences. However, I do feel that I should have simply accepted myself for the way I am. I should not have even tried secretly shaving off my body hair in the washroom with my dad's razor. For most of us, these aren't things we are equipped to deal with in adolescence. We just have to endure it, since in the end all we need is acceptance and self-love. I know that it isn't an inherent trait, but what helped me come to terms with it was when I stopped comparing myself with others. Learning about the journeys of people who don't necessarily follow the norms of society yet manage to flourish in their ventures was also inspiring. I understood that I don't need to change myself just to please others. If others could manage to live with that mindset and succeed, I could do it too!

On that note, it is nice to see people on social media slowly open up about their problems and talk things out. It is reassuring to know that we're all in this together. Moreover, it is encouraging to see that more people are sharing pictures of themselves without make-up or without a shave and without Photoshopping their pictures on social media these days. I feel the responsibility to act on this on my own social media accounts too. This is not to say that I can do this all the time, because I do still need to work and look a certain way to convince directors to give me appropriate roles. So even if my career is based on my appearance, at the end of the day, on social media at least, I try to portray who I am and what I look like without all the layers of make-up on me. For all the young girls who follow me, I hope that my transparency can reassure them that it is perfectly acceptable to look a certain way— any differences that they notice, whether in themselves or in others, need not be thought of as blemishes or imperfections, as we all have unique appearances. To add to that point, I need not be skinny or have 'meat' on my body in order to be successful, even if that has been the norm in the media industry for quite some time.

Getting back to the initial question, if your reason to lose fat or look a certain way is a conscious decision, then that is absolutely fine. However, I want to emphasize that no one should expect you to lose weight. No one has the right to tell me or you about what to do with our own bodies, especially with respect to losing weight (except our doctors maybe). Similarly, it is not realistic to shame yourself by constantly thinking about reaching an ideal weight, wanting to acquire a body that would look attractive in a bikini or even by comparing your physique with the toned bodies of others. Every person is unique—our genes, lifestyles and even our bodies are all different.

Unless you have the right motivation and attitude when it comes to fitness, you aren't going to enjoy the process and you're probably never going to be happy, even when you achieve your goals. Therefore, unless your reasons for wanting to lose weight are genuine, rather than driven by external factors, it'll be difficult to sustain the effort that goes into it.

However, if you decide to throw all other external reasons out of the window and prioritize getting healthy, strong and fit for your own sake, I welcome you with open arms.

A good thing to keep in mind when you want to lose excess body fat is to not have a specific time frame for it. Earlier, my haste to lose body fat became my biggest problem. For example, I would read in the newspaper about a certain actor gaining a lot of weight for a role in a new project, and consequently losing weight rapidly and getting very lean right afterwards for a second role in the same film. I would look at the pictures from when they were well built, and obsess over how they were able to change their physique so easily, wondering if I could do the same as well. But what I didn't understand back then was that the actor playing with their physicality might have had to rush the process due to a number of reasons. Primarily, they had to achieve it within that time frame due to the demands of the job. For instance, it might have been due to difficulties like the availability of the filming location or the availability of another actor on only a few dates. Whatever the reasons, the actor must have been following the protocols with guidance from experts in the field of fitness. They must have been constantly monitored throughout the process of attaining a certain physique, as well as after the performance to return their body to its regular form. For all the risks that they take, the production team would have agreed to spend enough for these experts as part of the actor's contract too.

We also tend to get carried away by the transformation pictures that we see. I am no exception to this, but while my posts about my clients' transformations on my Instagram profile include the before–after pictures, I put in the effort to explain in detail how the process of transformation had been achieved. What we normally fail to see in such pictures is an understanding of what has happened with the client. We see pictures from the first week and the fourth week and are charmed by the end result. We need to focus on the people themselves, whether they were given fat burners, how organically the transformation was achieved and so on. This is where the grass is green. Imagine having to maintain the same look throughout our lives. It is tough and requires a lot of discipline.

There is a very thin, imaginary line that separates being passionate about how we look and being obsessed about it. I have been on a rollercoaster ride when it comes to these two extremes for the longest time, and I am still not sure where I belong. Sometimes I have to consciously wrestle with and pull myself out of the weight of the expectation to look a certain way when it comes to my two careers—acting and fitness—both of which assign an importance to visual appeal. I have often thought about how easy my life would have been if I had chosen careers that did not place any demands on physical appearance. I have observed significant changes in my income when I don't look as attractive compared to how things are when I do. This is true not just me, but for the media fraternity. I know of a certain celebrity who follows the 'fasting and feasting' diet. For the first three days of the week, all they consume is a bowl of soup, some juice and herbal teas; on the next three days, they go all out and feast away. I'm not sure what happens on the seventh day.

Now, there is something known as 'mini cuts' which is nothing but a quick fat loss plan which bodybuilders use for competitions where they need to attain to a certain body fat percentage. Occasionally, when I need to look a certain way for a new role in a film that I do, or a photo shoot where I need to look sharp, I use a mini cut programme myself. It is usually for something that is time-bound, something that is planned out three to five weeks in advance. However, even this method is not suitable for a beginner. If you are an experienced health enthusiast, who has gone through the cycles of losing fat and maintaining your fat and muscle mass in the past, and you feel that you do have a profound degree of control over your body, then yes, this method can be used. The method needs to be followed to a T when it comes to eating. It is also an intense programme that combines strength training and cardio, which can energize you while you are on it. The most important thing one needs to keep in mind is to know when and how to ease up on the training regime on the days of your shoot in order to sustain it. It is also important to understand how to bring your metabolism and eating back to its normal state once you achieve your goals. Typically, the wrong way of going about any of these methods is to starve yourself because you are trying to reach a heavy calorie deficit and feel like giving in and eating everything that you can find. Your body needs to be gradually introduced to food during this time, and you need to de-load and take an active rest period for the next two weeks.

Trust me, it is impossible to 'naturally' have an hourglass figure. You either need to put in sustained and focused effort or follow an extremely unhealthy regime. So don't be fooled by the gorgeous bodies of your favourite film stars on screen. Nothing is ever that straightforward.

Most of us are not in a competition to lose fat on a strict timeline, and for those of you whose lives are not entirely dependent only on fitness or the way you look, I request you to do this slowly and steadily. Rushing the process is going to terribly backfire and take a toll on your body. Take it slow, take it easy, and learn to enjoy it and have fun while you're doing it. That is the only way to establish a lasting habit.

Here, I'd also like to broach the subject of eating disorders. I have heard of some models who have serious conditions like bulimia (eating and then purging by self-induced vomiting) and anorexia (starving and having an intense fear of gaining weight).[1]

---

[1] https://food.ndtv.com/health/8-famous-celebrities-who-battled-bulimia-1412998.

Please bear in mind that such extremities and eating disorders can have serious health consequences resulting in increased risk of heart failure, blood pressure, osteoporosis, kidney failure; they can also cause dehydration, gastric rupture, peptic ulcers, pancreatitis, depression, social anxiety, unstable moods, hypersensitivity, secretive behaviour and more. It is important to consult a medical practitioner and seek help in such situations as these are extremely dangerous and can lead to serious and severe psychological conditions.[2]

I am not an advocate of going under the knife to get your fat reduced due to a lack of willpower. Unless it is a medical requirement for your own health, this also tends to lead to other side effects, from what I have heard. The kinds of risks people take to lose weight are sometimes truly shocking! They all look fine on the outside, but behind the façade some people take enormous amounts of supplements every day, face staggering health conditions and constantly battle with trying to camouflage it all. Trust me, you do not want to go down the same path.

Looking amazing is one thing but feeling amazing and healthy is another. Looking good might give you a temporary high and boost your confidence in a superficial way, but that shouldn't be the main focus of getting fit. Looking good and feeling good must involve progressive work and changes to your overall lifestyle. Don't get confused between the two. In order to not fall off the wagon and having to regain what you

---

[2] See https://www.washcoll.edu/campus-community/health-and-counseling-services/counseling-center/eating-disorders/health-consequences.php; https://ohioline.osu.edu/factsheet/ED-1005-01-R11.

have lost, use sustainable practices. Remember that having the right mindset also helps influence the way you feel and look.

We will get to that, step by step!

Are you ready for the next exercise?

Exercise

Let us do something simple to rewire our brain. We are all so used to waking up in the morning, looking at ourselves in the mirror and then going 'Oh look at my face . . . OMG the dark circles'. Do you realize that this self-deprecation is ultimately toxic? It leads to an endless cycle of self-loathing for the rest of the day. What if you decided on three things now that you would say to yourself tomorrow morning in a kinder manner?

List them below.

1. _____

2. _____

3. _____

10

Exploring Your Body

Now that you've reflected on your reasons for wanting to lose fat, it's time to chalk out your goals. We all need to be clear about our fitness and health goals—what we want, what we're willing to give up and what we're not willing to let go of, in order to achieve them.

While it looks like the Instagram fitness influencers we see follow a specific 'secret diet' or 'secret workout module', from my personal story and learning from the experts around me, I can confidently tell you that the secret to getting fit, lean and strong is all the same—do it even if you don't like it.

If you're bored, do it. If you're lazy, do it anyway. If you're cranky, still do it.

'Do it' here refers to the discipline that you ought to have every single day to keep up with the routine of movement, physical activity, sleep and nutrition to meet the goals that you have in mind.

The most common fitness goals that I keep hearing over and over from clients who start out are:

- I want to get rid of my belly fat and love handles.
- I want to lose a certain number of kilograms or shed excess body fat.
- I want to regularize my period and stabilize any hormonal imbalances.
- I want to maintain my weight at the current range.
- I want to gain some weight (by adding muscle) without gaining excess fat in a particular spot.

Most of these can be achieved with the same principle: being on a calorie deficit plan, except for when you need to use a calorie surplus plan (I will explain these terms later in the book).

If you want to lose body fat, the best way to see changes would be to undertake a strength training plan for 3–4 days a week, combined with steady state cardio and movement consistently repeated for anywhere between 6–12 weeks without any distractions.[1]

The ideal training here which works well for me is the hypertrophy programme with 2–5 days of workouts a week, targeting one muscle group a day. What I enjoy in such a programme is that I feel it doesn't compromise on my muscles and helps me push for more power in training, increasing strength and calorie burn, which in turn aids in fat loss. Having used this method myself, I can suggest the same to you if this is your goal based on your body type, personal circumstances and so on.

---

[1] See https://www.verywellfit.com/cardio-and-weight-training-and-fat-loss-3498325.

So how long does it take to actually feel and even notice the changes in your body, in terms of inch loss or fat loss in a fat loss programme?

I figured that this really depends on several factors and varies from one person to another.

How strict are we on the calorie deficit/surplus plan?

Are we also going through something that is keeping us stressed, making us compromise on our sleep?

How are the workouts planned? Do they include too much of cardio?

This again can be further broken down to a Rate of Perceived Exertion Scale (RPES) in your strength and Perceived Effort Scale (PES) to understand the intensity of our activity while lifting weights or how spent we feel when we are working out. The more we transcend our limits and exert ourselves during the session, and the fewer breaks we take, the quicker and better will our results turn out to be.

Be informed that the amount of time it takes to lose fat can never be exactly estimated, and will vary from person to person, based on different factors like their genetics, height, weight, metabolism, sex and activity levels.

If you have a lot of fat to lose or you are starting out for the first time to lift weights, you will see rapid changes in your body. Our body doesn't like to get rid of fat since its duty is not to cater to our desires but to protect us and keep us alive even in life-threatening situations. As a result, it tries its best to store as much fat as it can. Therefore, over a period of time, after we have lost the initial chunk of excess fat, it is natural for the body to try to conserve fat and you will reach a plateau when it comes to further results.

You must have noticed that people who have been working out for a long time hardly progress with their lifts or muscle gains. For example, if you are a beginner and you lift 20 kg squats today on a barbell, I won't be surprised if you develop enough strength to be able to lift 30–35 kg by the end of the year! But in the case of a regular gym rat such as me, I would have to work really hard and will be extremely thankful if my body even gives me the strength to progress by 2–3 kg more by the end of each year. The same principle functions here—the body does not want to lose fat, but to accommodate the muscle gains it needs to get rid of fat, which works in our favour.

Just like undertraining, I find the other extreme of overtraining to be a problem with people who come to me for guidance these days. This is a more common problem with people as they age. As we age, our body takes more time to recover as well. You can't run a two-hour marathon in your forties and get ready for your training the very next day even if you were able to do that in your twenties! Resting is as important as working out in order to achieve the right results.

And here is the rub—whenever I have abused my body and pushed it over its limits, it has not worked in my favour, no matter how hard I exert myself. So I realized that if I am not giving my body enough time to rest and fully recover, instead of getting stronger, I'll simply be getting weaker, losing my metabolic activation and losing the muscles as well. We know that all of this is a recipe for disaster. So what I would love for you to take away from this is to be more worried about the quality of your workouts rather than the quantity. Adding more workouts will not ultimately help.

Body fat is like an obnoxious individual and no matter how much we do, if we do not put in time and effort as well as be patient, we cannot get rid of it; it will keep coming back.

Building muscle and lifting heavy weights require a calorie surplus or at least a calorie maintaining plan with more importance given to protein.[2]

In this case, if the goal is to increase strength, I would ideally focus on a strength training programme, but the difference in my training volume (number of sets and reps in each exercise) is the intensity of training and the weights I lift and the amount of rest time given to me in between sets. More importantly, my nutrition should be focused on a higher intake of protein than when I am on a calorie deficit plan to grow muscle in a surplus.

Now, here are a few things to keep in mind as you chalk out your fitness goals yourself:

1. Every body type is different—therefore, you should do
    what works best for you

Before planning a workout routine and diet, you need to understand your body in terms of its metabolism (more on that below), genetic factors, the amount of excess weight and fat deposits, the amount of calories you need and your macros (more on that in the chapter 'I Don't Eat Much but I Can't

---

[2] See https://www.healthline.com/nutrition/bulking#bottom-line. Also, https://www.trifectanutrition.com/blog/how-much-protein-do-i-need-to-build-muscle#:~:text=Bodybuilders%20and%20weightlifters%20have%20higher,average%20person%20or%20non%2Dlifter.

Lose the Fat'). Your lifestyle, age, sex and current food habits are also determining factors, like I said earlier.

It's important to get the consent and guidance of your physician before starting a new regimen, especially if you are pregnant, or if you have a specific health condition like thyroid, diabetes or blood pressure.

2.   Choose a workout you enjoy

Apart from the routine gym and High-Intensity Interval Training (HIIT) workouts, you could play a sport like cricket, tennis or badminton (making you accountable to the team you play with). You could also consider running or jogging outdoors (something I personally love—it's so simple, you just put on your gear and get out of the house!), yoga (for those of you who want to de-stress and calm your inner senses), Pilates, aerobics or Zumba (for those of you who enjoy dancing). You could even explore something skill-based, like learning a new martial art, a dance routine or even boxing—there are plenty of options.

3.   Know your metabolism

Each of us has that one friend who does not do much and yet effortlessly looks the same always, whereas we are the opposite type since we need to do a lot to keep up with them. Some people are just born with a good metabolism. This is what I'd mentioned about genetics playing a role! For the rest of us, we need to accept the metabolism that we are blessed (or not blessed) with, and work out a plan accordingly.

If you eat well and work out in a disciplined, optimal way for at least a year, and then take a fitness test with this friend of yours, you'll be surprised to find that you are the healthier one most of the time. I say this confidently because of my own experiences. A friend of mine once challenged me by saying that she would replicate what I'd achieved—instead of struggling through training, she'd get to my goals by doing absolutely nothing since she was just naturally blessed (I mean our proportionate figures here, in case you had any doubts!) Afterwards, we did a DEXA scan, which shows you the amount of fat, bone density and muscle mass in your body. The results, while rewarding for me, served as a wake-up call to make her realize that 'looking good' and 'being healthy' are two different things.

My point is that you might feel envious of people like them when you have to wake up and go on a jog while they don't do the same, or when you refuse an ice cream since you are being health conscious while they eat it without hesitation right in front of your eyes. However, you're more likely to be stronger and healthier by the end. More importantly, no two people are the same, so don't let such comparisons distract or discourage you.

Exercise

Knowing your fitness goals is the first step to understanding and achieving them. What are your top three fitness goals?

1. _____

2. _____

3. _____

11

My First Time

The first time you try out something is always special because of the element of curiosity in it.

For example, the first time you attended a mathematics class in school—you may have found it complicated and confusing, but probably still cherish the experience for so many other reasons.

Maybe it was the first (and only) time we were attentive in class because we were really curious about the subject (and hence didn't fall asleep).

Maybe it was the first time we met our first crush at school.

Maybe it was the first and last time we actually solved a maths problem correctly!

Like I said, the first time is truly memorable.

In this context, I am talking about the first time I worked out after making a realistic goal and getting a guided training programme for myself.

I still remember that I couldn't feel my body when I woke up the next morning. I couldn't even move, and every muscle ached and begged me not to get out of my bed. When I pushed myself and slowly and finally got up, I felt like I had been shocked in my quads (yes, it was right after a leg day).

Next, I had to take the steps to go downstairs. I cannot begin to tell you how painful that was! With each step, I cried out for my mom in pain. Then came the most difficult part—sitting at the breakfast table. I screamed so loudly that when I sat down and got up a few minutes later, the house started trembling a bit, and I felt like the walls were about to crack.

Am I saying this to warn you not to even attempt this? Absolutely not!

I am saying this because it is bound to happen when you start training seriously, and I want to prepare you for it to make you understand that this is how it is. This is a normal experience, for everyone. I don't want you to get scared when you experience something like this and shy away from the idea of doing an activity, if and when it happens. This exhaustion and pain that we are talking about here is known as Delayed Onset Muscle Soreness (DOMS) aka muscle soreness.[1]

Experienced by people who are new to fitness or have done an intense training session, this phenomenon occurs a certain period of time after you work out. It hits you out of nowhere, and you start to feel the pain.

The interesting thing about this kind of inflammation, which is good for us, is that:

---

[1] See https://www.nhs.uk/live-well/exercise/pain-after-exercise/#:~:text =DOMS%20typically%20lasts%20between%203,2%20days%20after%20 the%20exercise.

- Each one of us takes a different amount of time to experience this soreness. For some, it will occur within 8–12 hrs. For others, it can happen 24 hours later, and some even experience it after 48 hours of their training. I have personally experienced it usually 24–48 hours after my training.

- It is also a kind of a genetic response. This is to say that if you and I do the exact same kind of workout, I may feel the soreness whereas you may not feel anything at all. That has nothing to do with who worked out harder between the two of us. I used to get carried away and suffer from FOMO when, after a rock-solid training session, my gym mates would say they feel the soreness on their hamstrings and back muscles whereas I felt nothing. I would whine about this difference in our experiences until I learnt about this phenomenon!

- For some people, it's a strong and intense effect, while it affects others lightly. In my case, except for the first time when it was a sudden hit, this is normally a gradual and strange sensation in my body.

- Each muscle in our body works and responds differently. For example, my leg muscles often give me a good indication of the soreness after a heavy load session, but even when I have extensively worked on my traps or lats I never feel a similar soreness.

Overall, it is a kind of a good feeling, and that's how I'd take it. Why?

I know with soreness the indication is that the muscle at that spot has been worked to its optimum limit. The muscle then repairs and regrows after the damage, which is followed by muscle synthesis, which means that the new muscle formed will grow out to be stronger and tighter. It is a win-win situation, whether it is about looks, muscle definition or from a purely health perspective!

The takeaway here for you is that pain in any form is actually a good thing, and we should stop associating pain with negative feelings.[2] It is a part of our lives, and whether it shows up in fitness, your career, your relationships or in other areas, embracing it and working towards a solution to overcome the pain is the ideal plan—at least that's what works for me.

Again, balance it out folks! I myself have used soreness as a measure of a good workout in the past. After much training in a session, if I didn't feel any soreness at times, I would feel quite upset about it, thinking that I hadn't done a good job during the session.

Not feeling sore does not necessarily mean that you did not have a good workout session.

You simply have to remember to be your best while training as well as for the rest of the day, and leave the remainder for your body to handle, trusting that it knows what's best for you.

How do you know you are good to train while you are sore?

It depends on the intensity of the soreness that you feel, and the range of motion of the sore muscle.

---

[2] Do note that while some amount of pain is normal, excessive pain may require medical assistance.

If it feels too difficult to even move the muscle, you should relax and take some time off until you feel okay.

If the soreness is merely a tingling in your muscles, something that is not too intense, just go ahead with your session on the next day after a solid warm-up to take you through the session.

Do you know what would help you recover faster?

1. Drinking lots of water
2. Yoga stretches and foam rolling
3. A gentle, full-body deep conditioning massage

Normally, if you prefer concrete training plans, the workouts should be planned in a way such that we don't tire out the same muscle continuously. It is also good to take a gap for at least a day or two before getting back to the muscle group we finished training with.

Over time, the soreness you have will disappear as your body starts to become habituated to the kind of workouts you do. As they say, 'no pain, no gain'!

Monitoring your progress and being aware of your condition is a big part of what one should do when we start taking care of ourselves.

Also, be sure to monitor your pain and sense the difference between soreness and a muscle spasm or injury. If the pain is excruciating and intolerable, and it doesn't go away after 3–4 days, it might be a spasm or an injury, which would require medical attention.

Talking about soreness and workouts, this was one of the earliest routines I started out with which made me have fun

ılso resulted in the right amount of soreness for
ıfter the session. Do it whenever you want to!

your first and last name, and do this quick
Alphabet workout:

(This is a workout that you can do on your own if you are
someone who has had exposure to HIIT training before.
Otherwise, do it with the guidance of someone who can
spot and help you out. The exercises are simple but effective,
and can be done without any weights or with lightweights
depending on your experience and fitness levels.)

A: 10 Burpees	N: 15 Donkey Kicks
B: 15 Push-ups	O: High Knees—45 seconds
C: 20 Reverse Lunges	P: 15 V-ups
D: Plank—2 minutes	Q: 15 Split Squats
E: 50 Jumping Jacks	R: 20 Glute Bridges
F: 20 Leg Raises	S: 15 Step-ups
G: 30 Ab Crunches	T: 10 Alternating Toe-touch Crunches
H: 30 Star Jumps	U: Up and down the staircase—5 times
I: 25 Squats	V: 20 Jump Squats
J: 15 Triceps Dips	W: 20 Bicycle Crunches
K: 20 Mountain Climbers	X: 25 Calf Raises
L: Wall Sit—1 minute	Y: 20 Fire Hydrants
M: Side Planks—1 minute for each side	Z: 15 Inchworms

12

How I Got My Mojo Back

I have always been the type of person who has been drawn to doing things outside the norm. I have made a few career related decisions that have helped me stand out—for example, I studied visual communication, then I was a television anchor, then I did modeling and took part in a beauty pageant, became a radio jockey and an actor soon afterwards, followed by becoming a powerlifter, YouTuber and an author. Recently, I have also become a fitness entrepreneur and a health coach. So far, there has been no one in my family who has pursued any of these careers. I could not use any family member as an example to convince my parents each time I decided on a new job. It just flowed this way for me because of the support from my parents. At the end of the day, they wanted me to be happy and feel accomplished, and had full faith in my decisions. That is what gave me the courage and discipline to keep going.

In spite of this working for me, I know that this trajectory isn't easy for every girl out there, even now. More often than not, the girl who hangs out with the boys and plays sports in school is judged and seen as an example of what girls aren't supposed to do. This is sadly the majority mindset that our society has when it comes to women's physicality.

When I used to think the same way, I could never imagine that I would become a powerlifter at some stage in my life. I had hardly ever lifted weights nor been actively involved in any outdoor sports, either during my school life or my time at college.

The reason I fell in love with powerlifting was that while I had no major female powerlifters with me in the arena, the little number of women I saw were all so focused on their performance and their health that they really didn't care about how they looked. That, to me, was extremely empowering. Having been in a career where society required me to look a certain way and be 'ladylike', and at a time when I was suffering from eating disorders, low self-esteem and was never feeling comfortable and satisfied with who I was and how I looked, I felt that this change of focusing from how my body looked to what my body could do would be a very positive thing for me.

Until that point, from my perspective, exercise was for the sole purpose of burning off the calories from whatever I had eaten—that was clearly self-destructive. After ten years of pleasing society and playing by the norms, my breakthrough moment was when I could simply decide to do whatever made me satisfied. I could lift, fuel my body enough for it to perform well and could unabashedly look whatever way I would on the path to reaching my fitness goals. That was when I began to feel comfortable in my own skin, and I could embrace the ideas of self-love and self-confidence.

Let me tell you the story of how it all started. In the past, when I was working with my trainer Jyotsna, she saw my passion for working out, be it cardio, HIIT or any other kind of exercise, and she broached the idea that I should attempt powerlifting. Back in 2017, I knew nothing of it. I just became curious and started watching videos on YouTube of international powerlifters to understand what she really meant. At that point, I desperately wanted a change of things just to feel better, so I agreed to her proposal. We did focussed training sessions for hardly a week, before my first powerlifting competition that involved only the bench press. I had no expectations and was just curious to see how it works, and hardly practised the bench press at that time because I was scared it would fall on my head (after watching an old Vadivelu comedy where the bar would land on his face whenever the spotter let it go). I did a 1 RM of 32.5 kg on the bench at the competition and was awarded first place, without even knowing that I was already strong enough to compete with other women in my weight range at that point! From then to now, I have graduated to about 1 RM of 45 kg without any dedicated regime on the bench and I attribute this to my muscle growth over the year.

Training and preparing for powerlifting competitions is entirely different from the regular training that we do for fat loss. When I was completely new to lifting weights, I could see what we call 'beginner gains' in my body. This would often be something like an additional bit of muscle that helped me lift more. This helped me appreciate the work and activity I was doing. After this, everything stalled in the area of muscle gains. This is very common, and it was unrealistic of me to try to increase the weight I lifted out of desperation. The biggest challenge for a powerlifter is fatigue and the ability to manage it. Unlike in a fat loss programme, where you push through that fatigue and can go train even with all the soreness, handling fatigue in powerlifting, by giving the body enough time to rest and recover before reattempting a lift in squat or bench press or dead lift, is extremely crucial. Thus, I would do quick sets of small reps, but hit the muscle groups every other day to keep pushing the score on the weights. I still remember the funny walk because of the solid burn on my glutes after my powerlifting squat days. Powerlifters also tend to save up all the energy for the heavy lifts. We do not, in this time, focus on the cardio sessions as much as we would otherwise. I also had to eat a lot of carbohydrates and high protein to build more muscle and recover well and push myself more with each session.

Again, this was an epiphany for me—if I was too focused on the aesthetics, or even getting physically stronger at the cost of neglecting my health, it was impossible to progress. Therefore, this path of pushing harder and harder while not eating healthily was not something I could afford to do in this phase.

Even now when I think about it, I distinctly recall the strong scent of a popular pain-relief gel that filled the rooms where groups of powerfully built men were doing insanely heavy lifts. I will never forget the look on their faces when I walked in—I was one of the few women entering the powerlifting arena, and that too, I was from the entertainment industry, so nobody was expecting me there. After the initial murmurs, greetings and checking to see if I was the real Ramya they had seen on television, the crowd, filled with a majority of men, supported me all the way. Being a newbie, I wasn't completely sure of the rules of the competition. Some of them guided me with the formal procedures on how to wait for instructions before doing the lift, gave me tips to warm up, warned me what not to do to avoid disqualification and helped me look the part for the competition.

As nervous as I was, I wanted to ace this—both for myself and for those who believed in me. After my weigh-in, I ate a banana and a few dates that I had carried along, did my warm-up and waited for my turn.

When my name was called, I went to my spot, focused my entire mind and energy on the challenge and visualized myself lifting the weight. I was fully conscious of the adrenaline rush inside me and soaked in the cheers from the amazing audience around me. And then . . . I just lifted. I did it!

Almost every single person—even the brawny, well-built and adorable men in the room—hooted and cheered for me in full force every time my name was called. I could see that they all really wanted me to succeed. Hundreds of strong men came together to encourage a woman to prove her worth in powerlifting, and celebrate her strength and ability—how often do we see something like that? I loved it! That was something I had craved for all my life, and it finally happened.

The whistles and thundering applause that erupted around me dazed me for a while. It gave me a renewed sense of hope about life. I knew that this was a turning point, and that my life was about to change for the better. It was exactly the reassurance and validation I needed to regain my lost confidence and zest for life. It was my medicine to heal.

This was also the phase when I was feeling particularly stagnated in life and with all the jobs that I was engaged in. I had been anchoring from the time I was at school and I had been exposed to a lot of shows, events and different formats of hosting, from a corporate show to awards nights. I started feeling that I needed some change in my life, or at least a break of some sorts. I was on a quest for looking at what was the next thing I could do in life that I could be really good at. This, in turn, led to a lot of trial and error. I tried starting a celebrity management company, a bakery, doing casting for films and becoming a full-time Bharatnatyam dancer, but nothing really clicked at the time.

There was a certain amount of self-doubt initially, while I was on the path of powerlifting and trying to figure out if the world of fitness is where I belong. When there are a lot of eyes on you, there are more expectations, and there is also the pressure to perform well in a competition that you participate in, whether it is at a district or state level. With greater exposure, potential for people to both like and dislike you also increases. When I had just started out on this journey in the fitness world by sharing videos of myself exercising on social media, realizing the sheer number of people who wrote a lot of discouraging criticism and wanted to see me fail (added to the failed relationship that I was slowly recovering from) was crushing. These comments were either about my appearance, pointing out that I was starting to look like a man, or they were falsely concerned about my health, suggesting that I would need to be hospitalized soon or suffer from a major accident because of all the heavy lifting. I was struggling to realize that their hate was a manifestation of their jealousy, which made their actions and comments justified to them since they believed that I was acting wrongly (not being their version of what a woman is 'supposed to be').

This was adding to my already prevalent performance anxiety when it came to doing my best. Every time I went to the competition arena, that desperation to perform better than the last time was emotionally gruelling for me to handle. I had addressed several thousands of people onstage or talked to the camera knowing that millions of people would watch me while I worked as an anchor. However, this was vastly different, as I was alone in an arena performing a physical task, with everyone's eyes on me. Their gaze was much closer to me than onstage or even through a camera. Seeing others perform in front of my eyes, either doing better than me or failing due to a silly error like not following the command in a flow, was making me insecure about how I would handle the task in those few seconds when I was supposed to be in the spotlight.

There are no shortcuts when it comes to fear and anxiety, and facing those fears head-on was an important lesson I learnt at the time. I had to become thick-skinned and stop beating myself up over what other people thought about me whenever I was criticized for uploading a video of me lifting weights. Over time, I thought less about the comments and more about self-acceptance, and the road from that point on has been great.

This has been a great phase of my life—powerlifting made me realize my true potential and pushed me in the right direction, towards what I was meant to do to make my life meaningful. Though the life of a celebrity gave me fame, attention and accolades, it is my health coaching in the last two years that has made me feel like I am adding value to others' lives. Be it a teenager who tells me she joined my programme, which led to her period cycles becoming regular, or a woman struggling to get pregnant, who comes and holds my hands and thanks me for the support I had given her to help her knock off the excess fat which was hindering her pregnancy— all these experiences make me feel extremely satisfied in this line of job, more than everything else that I do. All of this is thanks to my powerful messages in my journey of powerlifting! And yes, I strongly believe that there is a supreme power which is guiding me at every step and pushing me forward by overcoming every challenge that I encounter.

13

Balancing Being a Cheerleader and Game Spoiler

The hardest part about following a diet is getting accepted by the people closest to us. We often find it more uncomfortable to explain to people that we are on a diet than actually following the diet itself. In the past, I have felt too embarrassed to even tell a friend that I am on a certain regime and need to get more disciplined to get into better shape. Why does this happen?

I used to worry that they would make fun of me once they found out, discourage me, be unsupportive or even share these private details with others and embarrass me more. In some rare cases, they would be too excited and offer unsolicited advice, share articles with me and even send messages in the morning reminding me to not drink my coffee with sugar. Their suggestions, which might have worked for them, would be shared too often and make me feel too overwhelmed and uncomfortable. I mostly find that the people around us either tend to be overenthusiastic or have no reactions or comments at all; there is hardly a middle ground. To understand that our health goals are very personal and to approach them in a sensitive way is what is needed, and there is a thin line between ignoring the communication altogether and showing that you care for someone who is attempting to do something new with their health and body.

Not judging others' decisions to embark on a fitness journey, and cheering them up with a 'hope you had a good workout today' or 'it's nice to see you so committed to your goals' or 'I am happy for the choice that you have made to take care of yourself' seems like a nice start. Making fun of the way they exercise, laughing and mocking them when they make some changes to their eating habits and forcing them to lose weight is definitely the wrong way to go about it.

If you're a family member or a close friend who knows a lot about the person, certain words of encouragement like 'You have lost oodles of weight', or 'You have downsized a lot' go a long way for someone who has a long-term plan for losing body fat and getting fit. Previously, I used to think that noticing that someone had gotten slimmer than before and appreciating it was a good thing. But one day, I started thinking and considered if that person did not choose to lose that weight in the first place. What if they were ill or were suffering from some kind of depression which had physical effects in the form of weight loss? Therefore, after that day, unless I coach a client who has a certain goal or I know a certain friend who would definitely be happy when I mention their weight loss, I hold my horses and simply don't make any remarks about anyone's body.

Now, the family members who live with you will be extremely crucial in your journey to meet your health goals. They can completely make it or break it for you.

I'd compare starting a new diet to the kind of feeling you have when you change schools and enter your new class on your first day. You have no clue how things will go, and there's a sense of unease that haunts you till you settle down.

My mom was born and raised in this little town called Mannargudi near Thanjavur. To this day, she advocates the idea of eating high carb refined foods like *pazhayadu* (fermented rice), pongal, poori, *kozhakattai* (steamed rice flour dumpling) and vada every day for breakfast. Her reasoning is '*Kalla thinaalaalum serikura vayasu idhu*' (When you're young, even if you eat a stone you'll be able to digest it).

I agree that *pazhayadu* is awesome and has some fantastic benefits, and I don't dislike carbohydrates either. I love eating idli, dosa, dal, *adai*, *pesarattu*, millets, sattu (porridge) and oats. Having said that, I think that our work and lifestyle should determine the amount of carbs we consume. Also, I do not consume refined carbs and starchy vegetables at all, as it just doesn't sit well with my gut. In our current situation, I feel that we need to make small changes from how our ancestors ate back in the day, when they were physically hyperactive, to the present when we are all leading a sedentary, gadget-driven lifestyle. That realization alone will help us stop going wrong nutritionally.

So, to fit into the same clothes and maintain a healthy lifestyle, you must first understand how to plan your eating habits based on your personal situation. Let me warn you about the challenges you might face if you are the only one in your entire family who is on a certain diet regime:

First, your family will look at you like you are an alien who is doing something wrong to the world by trying to eat right! After this, stage two may include taunts and discouragement every time you consciously make an effort to eat a balanced meal—practising portion control, politely refuse the oil-soaked, deep-fried potato roast, or not eating that sugar and ghee-loaded *sakkarai* pongal. If surpassing the temptation of the food your family consumes and working on your self-control is one big challenge in itself, making them respect your choice of not having the food is another difficult task! In stage 3, you'll be attacked with constant comparisons of how you used to eat as a child (as if you had much of a choice back then!) and how you have become incorrigible now!

They might also point out how they eat whatever they want and nothing has gone wrong with them. Remember the word bio-individuality when they say this. One person's food is the other's poison, and their lifestyle and yours is not the same. We need to agree to that.

The third month onwards is when they'll start accepting— or rather, putting up with—your regime and discipline. By this time, they'll have realized that there is no use making so much noise anyway since they don't believe you are going to listen to them.

The roadblocks you will face with friends and colleagues are a whole different ball game. Friends who invite you to dinners, birthday parties or weddings will get terribly offended by the changes you've decided to make. Rather than understand or appreciate the effort I was trying to make, most people around me would ridicule and discourage me by saying things like 'You don't enjoy your life enough' or 'You're pushing it too much'. They would ask questions like 'Why are you wasting time working so hard on yourself?' or 'What is the point of all this!?'

We tend to associate getting healthy with something that is not fun and requires heavy sacrifice. I beg to differ. A well-crafted strategy for attaining your goal would ideally have everything that you want. You can have your cup of coffee or tea, you can have that slice of pizza over the weekend and you can do an activity that you enjoy. Remember it is not that one cup of tea or a bite of pizza that changes everything, but what you do for the rest of the day after that. All you need is some structure and planning. In fact, I am having a slice of chocolate cake now while I am writing this out to you.

If you are a complete party maniac or a social butterfly, trying to stay fit is very difficult. The fact that I wasn't one definitely helped me put my head back down and stay on track. Firstly, it saved me from having my focus and discipline being depleted. I wouldn't be able to resist my temptations and would give in at that moment, eat all I wanted, feel bad later in the night leading to further eating due to my guilt, and kick-start the whole plan again the next day 'from the beginning'. This is what happened the few times I had to step out for a family event while being on a regime. I realized much later that I don't have to give up out of frustration or go back to restart everything for one bad day of eating. Simply being mindful of what I eat on the days that follow and increase the training intensity by a bit is sufficient.

After all, mindset training is similar to training a muscle. Initially, we will all fail at it, but handling it properly and keeping our mind alert eventually helps us focus on the bigger goal.

It worked out better after a few attempts of me staying by myself and not letting distractions come my way while I was on a programme, if I was extremely determined to get good results. Later, when I started seeing some physical changes, and then began to show my face at weddings and public events again, the compliments and reactions felt very rewarding, and gave me the confidence to keep going. By then, I had the mindset to be able to take decisions about whether or not I wanted to indulge people's requests at a given moment without getting hassled. This is a better strategy for me these days. However, if I do not have any specific goals, I just enjoy the little diet breaks, since I am comfortable with knowing that it may take a while for me to see the results of my training.

My mantra when it comes to mindset training is this: Not everyone will support us in the process, but everyone will celebrate us when we reach our goal. In other words, the world needs to see your success to celebrate you.

My Top Five Cheerleaders in My Fitness Journey

1. My fans, my followers, the people who make me feel motivated to not fail them and keep on going. It is those positive messages, comments and emails that you send to me, which wake me up on the days when I feel particularly dispirited. I love you all, and no matter how many times I say this, it won't be enough!

2. My two partners and friends in the gym, Venkatesh Kannan and Deepak. They not only constantly keep on encouraging me, saying how my look and muscle definition keep progressing over the years compared to

when I started, but they also spot me, push me to brace up and lift more. Thank you guys; you have been a great support to me, especially on days when I lacked the motiviation to head to the gym!!

3. My mother and father—they secretly share the details about my strength and the discipline I practise with other relatives and friends. They talk about it with pride when discussing these details with others, but also keep me grounded when they're talking to me. With my uncles and *athais* asking me to coach them on their health recently, my mom's happiness has no limits in this area.

4. My fitness role models Sam Sweeney and Senada Greca, who inspire me each day with their posts on Instagram and get me excited to go to the gym. They don't know that they inspire me and are my cheerleaders, but I hope they find out once this book is published! Every time I get a reply from them on Instagram, I just can't stop smiling for the rest of the day!

5. Me. I am my own cheerleader, and I pull myself up to get things done, even on the days when I don't want to get out of the bed in the morning.

So that was my list. Write out who your top five cheerleaders are in the list below:

1. _____
2. _____
3. _____
4. _____
5. _____

14

Ownership and Partnership

The most important thing I've learnt is that you can never make people adapt to a healthy way of life just through words.

Like I explained it earlier in my own case, as parents, it is our responsibility to not entirely restrict indulgences and help the child grow around a healthy food environment. While this is partly done with the kind of food we cook and feed them, it is also impactful for the child to see our own food choices and eating habits. How would it be acceptable to limit the food that growing children can eat and advise them to reduce their fried food and chocolate intake when they see us constantly snacking on savouries and brownies and cupcakes? Pointing fingers at a child, at that impressionable age, can become more of a trigger of mental disturbance. It might not be my place to offer parenting advice, but this is an observation that I've made from how common this is among several of my own friends. They keep alternating between the extremes when it comes to feeding their kids. I totally understand how difficult it is to execute this, but trust me, it is definitely manageable—I have already seen some parents nailing this!

To this day, I have never tried to impose my own diet and fitness regimes on my parents.

They have rice for brunch, dosa, idli or pongal as a snack, and rice again for dinner; I have a smoothie or an omelette for breakfast, a varied lunch each day that is high on protein and veggies, nut butter or a fruit as a snack and a salad, followed by soup for dinner. On some days I just eat two big meals, and on other days I eat three.

I've also noticed that my parents are both extremely active, and this kind of an eating plan works for them given the eating pattern that they have always been used to. The food that they eat has no processed ingredients in them, and they also never compromise on their daily walks. I have hardly ever seen either my dad or my mom eat food prepared outside, and even on the rarest of occasions when we do go out for a meal or I order in, they don't enjoy having it. For them, food has to be made fresh and cooked in a very simple manner.

They don't go overboard with the eating portions either. Although my mom still hasn't come to terms with how I eat, she stopped complaining about it when she began to notice the kind of strength my body has picked up in the last few years (thanks to my adequate protein intake now)—for instance, I can lift up the gas cylinder or help her load and unload packages in the storeroom. She's also realized that I have developed a strong immune system and don't fall as sick as I used to earlier (touch wood). With all these benefits, plus the compliments she gets from her friends about my fitness abilities and the content on my YouTube channel, she lets me be in peace. Since I have also understood their lifestyle, the system and discipline that they have adapted to when it comes to eating, I see no reason to try and change it.

Having said that, it is still important to have a rational discussion with your family before you begin pursuing your fitness goals. You need to help them understand how important this is to you. If constantly seeing junk food in the kitchen or on the dining table is weakening your will, tell them that you'd prefer to keep all their junk food stored away. If they frequently invite you to join them for dinners or lunches, politely decline once in a while. Alternatively, you could volunteer to choose the dining locales yourself, so that you can find a restaurant or cafe with some healthy options. These days, every restaurant has a set of healthy items on the menu or, at the very least, some soups and salads to choose from. Worst-case scenario, you could always request the chef or manager to make you a serving that's not drenched in oil and masala. If your family likes to order in most of the time, cook your own meals at home instead.

However, it never hurts to have someone workout alongside you, and that can be some added fun and accountability as well. You don't need to have all your family members join you, but having at least one buddy outside or within your home can make a huge difference. It could be your spouse, partner, mom, dad, a sibling or a friend. When I was in the tenth grade, I used to love taking walks in the morning with my best friend Sadhana, who lived a street away from my home, on the days before our exams. We used to wake up as early as possible to revise for our exams, and at around 6 a.m., Sadhana and I would start walking together for about thirty minutes to just get some fresh air and discuss our doubts on subjects we weren't sure of. We did not know then that we were also performing a physical activity, but it used to be something we always looked forward to.

Here's the special thing about workout buddies: I've found that all of mine have become my best friends over time. While I initially met most of my workout partners today at the gym, our bonding time slowly expanded over jogs, badminton sessions, going on food trails and even pilgrimages together. We'd also share interesting workouts, recipes with healthy macros and articles related to health and fitness with each other, as well as have healthy challenges among us. We'd compete to see how many burpees we could get done in a minute. We'd push one another for an extra round of AMRAP workout[1] or an ab finisher. There are so many days when I don't feel quite motivated to go do a workout, but the company of my friends is the only reason that pushes me to show up. Once I reach the gym, my motivation rapidly increases—I often start exercising with greater intensity and even push my friends along with me too! This applied even during the full lockdowns over the last two years. We all smartly invested in a couple of dumb-bells and then it became a habitual nightly routine for us to plan on a common time for the workout. I'd wake up, get on a Zoom call and start the workout that I had prepared the previous night, while one of them played some music from their playlist to get us pumped up to train. These would often be a one-hour session of solid lifts, fun and laughs in between and death by R's training in the end. In fact, we were so addicted to this that we never compromised on the training for any reason,

---

[1] AMRAP stands for 'As many rounds as possible'.

and we ultimately completed more workouts virtually than what we would have done if we had to meet in person. Also, since I was so used to the comfort of many kinds of equipment around me and a coach to push me to progress, I would not have done my workouts this religiously during the lockdown if I did not have my accountability partners.

It is both uplifting and motivating to be part of a community held together by a common interest in fitness. I do understand that you can't force someone to join you for workouts, and the interest must be mutual. There are other things as well, like their work schedules and syncing up their free time with yours. You know what I would suggest in this case? Join an online community or a Facebook group that is dedicated to fitness and health. There are hundreds of groups online, and you need to choose the one that resonates with you.

During the lockdown, I opened up an online live group workout module as part of my health coaching, calling it the 'Transform with Ramya' (TWR) series. It started as a trial of an everyday live virtual training programme for about 4 weeks. My only intention of curating this was to help people stuck at home to wake up with something to look forward to each day, get some activity done, clear their heads and reduce their anxiety. I was also offering free workout sessions on my Instagram account 'StayFitWithRamya' (SFWR), and every time I did one, more than 100 members would line up to get access to the Zoom session (which had its limits set to only 100 participants then)!

I had about fifty people signing up for this programme, and as much as I was delighted with the participation, I wasn't sure how many would turn up consistently, given that it was something very new that I was trying out too. All of the participants were added to a WhatsApp group so that we could communicate and make announcements efficiently. This is where I also discovered the gains behind a solid community.

This WhatsApp group had a diversified audience who lived in different countries, different cities, belonged to different age groups, spoke different languages and so on. But the one thing they were excited about was what they had in common—someone similar to them who wanted to give it a shot at getting healthy. They shared motivational quotes with each other, recipes they cooked at home during the lockdown, helped each other by sharing links for where to get the right shoes to train, discussed topics like whey protein and how it had impacted them, how they felt after a session, and also gradually started checking in on those who were absent. It was like a solid fitness army that I was building through my programme, and I was overjoyed! From getting requests for songs to be played during a session, to making plans to meet up post the lockdown and adding each other on Instagram, this network that I put together was only getting bigger and better! We almost had a farewell when we finished the programme, and everyone who had enrolled was asking over and over again about when my next programme would begin. This first edition also taught me the most important purpose behind what my role as a health coach should be. I like to help people achieve their goals, build a community for them and keep it running for them happily ever after. The second edition began right after the humongous response to the first one, and now there is no looking back on TWR group programmes! I even did little barbecues, coffee meetups and met my community in cities that I travelled to, after giving prior notice to them.

I now feel like I have friends all over the country, and many of my clients are Indian women living abroad. The bigger my SFWR community grows, the more fulfilled I feel with regard to my purpose as a health coach. Maybe someday, I can plan customized retreats for this happy, healthy community. They can relax, have fun and heal themselves physically, mentally, spiritually and holistically while they're on this vacation. That's the end goal for me. We shall achieve it someday!

Joining an online training programme or a gym membership is never a problem that I see among people who want to start anew. What you do to adapt to the programme and the methods you use to sustain it help to build the right habits for you to continue with the programme.

Seek the support that you need in whatever form that you want. For some of you, it can be your partner rolling next to you in the bed, while for others it can be someone random whom you have never met before. Regardless of who or what you seek, this community and its benefits are extremely valuable.

Benefits of having a workout buddy:

1. Accountability. They will help you stay committed to your workout.
2. They will help you step out of your comfort zone and push you when you're slacking.
3. Having someone to work out with is always fun.
4. You'll always have someone to talk to about your workout and diet and will be motivated to stay healthy.
5. It will strengthen the emotional bond between you and your buddy.

15

Meal Prepping

Working women often talk about how meal prepping has been a lifesaver. India hasn't quite bought into meal prepping in a big way yet.

First and foremost, meal planning and meal prepping are completely different.

How do you plan a meal?

Understand your schedule first. What are your weekdays and weekends like?

If you have a meal plan, you can split your macros into how many meals you plan to have in a given day.

Next, analyse your body. When do you feel the hungriest? Are you someone who gets hungry in the morning and needs to eat breakfast, or are you someone who can't look at food early in the morning? Plan the meals based on your own timings and needs.

It can even be as simple as eating five hard-boiled eggs that I decide to have after my time at the gym. Because I had mentally pre-planned to have them and had boiled the eggs already, I would not make poor food choices anymore just because I worked all day long and had no time to cook and eat healthy. This is the single most important tip I normally give out to those who stay in hostels and say that they are having a hard time cooking and yet want to eat healthy.

Do I do all of this every day? No, not anymore. I make a mental plan every morning, or on the night before if I have to travel or have a shoot the following day. I try to stick to these plans most of the time. I settle on a flexible routine, where I don't necessarily take three hours on a Sunday to meal prep but I definitely plan things out.

With a lot of my clients who suffer from not hitting their macros[1] or having inadequate protein intake, meal prepping has been a lifesaver. Meal planning can begin after you get comfortable making your food choices for a decent amount of time.

If you're about to say, 'But, oh! I don't have time for meal prepping on a weekend', you would just make me roll my eyes. If this is important enough to you, you can cut down on an hour of scrolling on social media on a lazy Sunday and devote it to this to make your life smoother for the rest of the week.

---

[1] Macros, short for macronutrients. In broader terms the most important ones are carbohydrates, fats and proteins. Each person's required macros would depend on their weight/height/lifestyle and body goals at that point. See https://www.sclhealth.org/blog/2018/10/what-are-macros-and-why-should-i-be-counting-them/#:~:text=Well%2C%20%E2%80%9Cmacro%E2%80%9D%20is%20short,fat%20that%20you're%20consuming.

Meal prepping is a practical and ideal solution for many situations you might encounter, and it has plenty of benefits too:

- If you live with your family at home, but you are the only one working towards a health goal, cooking separate meals for yourself every day can be difficult and impractical. When you meal prep every Sunday for the week ahead, both cooking and eating become simpler for you.
- If you are also cooking for your entire family, having your own meals prepped not only saves time, but also gives you the comfort of eating your food whenever you want to, possibly before or after you've cooked for the rest of the family. This way, you'll avoid a situation where you hungrily go into the kitchen and satiate yourself by eating whatever's in front of you—saving you from potentially bigger portions and unhealthier food.
- Meal prepping doesn't mean that you make and eat the same food over and over every day. It helps in planning ahead and encourages you to creatively use the ingredients that you have, adding variety to your meals.
- Apart from all of this, it saves a lot of money (fewer trips to the grocery store), reduces food wastage, and helps you eat out less too.

Coming to the basics of meal prepping, there is the lazy approach—only prepare certain meals a day (which I also call 'struggle meals'). If I prepare my dinner, which is usually the meal that I indulge myself with after a tiring day, I focus on prepping just that one single meal and make a dinner plan for myself.

What do you need for meal prepping?

A kitchen scale, some cups and spoons with varied measurements, some bowls for storage, and you're all set.

Measure your carbs and measure your portions of protein—this would be of great help when you're logging and tracking your food for whatever your goal is. Also, when you start doing this, you will soon learn how much a tablespoon of butter looks like, or what 100 grams of raw rice is—this will eventually help you gain an intuition for measurements later on, when you can simply eyeball the food to glean its nutritional value, macros and calories. Imagine how cool that would be. So include your toppings, spreads and condiments, and understand the portions you add into your food while prepping.

Meal prepping can simply be cutting all your vegetables in advance, or cutting and dry roasting them with spices on a non-stick pan and keeping them in a ready-to-use masala or dip form. Meal prepping isn't something boring like some of you might think it to be. Switch it up! If your gravy is done, change the veggies in it. If your veggies are too similar, change the texture of your seasoning and so on. Just get creative with your cooking if you are someone who likes variety. You could also semi- or fully cook your meal and stock it in the refrigerator, then just heat it up before you eat it. It's all up to you.

I am a big proponent of cooking things simply while doing meal prep and seasoning it later at the time of eating it if I am at home, or in the morning right before packing it if I have to go outside.

The reason is that there are chances for the food to change its texture and taste, and if it becomes dry you need to add the oil again, or add herbs or cheese which will lead to the macros changing and your calories getting higher again. So why not just cut it, boil it, grill it or bake it—whatever you normally do—and store it so that you can season its taste later? Another thing I notice is that with meal prepping, everything lasts longer without seasoning on it. So, if you are trying to cook your chicken or paneer, simply cook it plainly in the tawa, oven or grill, and store in the fridge or freezer. This is a nifty meal prep trick. You can defrost it later, and quickly heat it and add your spices or condiments and eat away.

Now let me take each macronutrient and break down a few options for you to meal prep in advance.

Let's start with protein.

- Lean cuts of fish, chicken or any other grass-fed meat that you prefer (please grill these for optimal benefits).
- Protein powders that can be added to overnight oats and chia puddings (even stirring it in water and having it is good enough).
- Boiled eggs can be stored in the refrigerator and can be eaten at any time as a snack! For those who avoid the yolk owing to the cholesterol, I normally suggest a 4:1 ratio (for every 4 egg whites, you can have 1 yolk), or if you don't want to waste the egg yolks, just get the egg white fluids that are available in the markets these days.
- Tofu, soya and tempeh are handy too. Chia seeds, flax seeds and oats are good options to use for meal prepping as well.

Next, let's look at carbohydrates.

- Include all the green vegetables, carrots, beetroots, squashes, leafy greens, sweet potatoes, radishes, pumpkins and colourful veggies.
- Fruits that are low in sugar—apples, small bananas, berries, guavas, pears, black grapes, papayas, watermelons, plums, cherries, etc.
- Then include all the lentils, legumes, dals and pulses.
- Also, you can use non-refined sources of rice, millet, edamame, sourdough, quinoa, pasta, sattu and whole wheat. You can do anything for carbs, as long as you avoid processing it and keep the portions in control.

Let's move on to fats. You can use:

- Nut butters
- Avocados
- Nuts
- Greek yoghurt
- Buttermilk
- Low-fat cheese or low-fat paneer

Apart from these, you can list down the foods you personally enjoy and find substitutes for it. For example, if you like chocolates opt for 70 per cent and above dark chocolate. Some of you might like peanut *chikki*—organic laddoo would be a better alternative. If you drink hot beverages twice a day, see if you can replace the sugar with brown sugar, jaggery, cane sugar or stevia. All of this depends on your goals and your macro allowances. These substitutes are not mandatory, but just suggestions to allow for a healthier lifestyle.

Again, I am getting back to the idea that eating healthy need not be boring. When you go grocery shopping, all you need to pick up is two to three options for protein, carbs and a wide range of colourful veggies—that's it. It is then a matter of switching up the macro sources each day when you are making your dishes.

How do you combine these into meals after meal prepping?

My general suggestion is that for every meal distribute having half a cup of the carbs, three-fourth cups of protein and a minimum of one to one and a half cup of veggies. Fat is usually used in cooking, so I personally don't think it needs to be included separately. I will discuss exact portions and how to calculate them in the upcoming macros calculation chapter.

These days, there are also some fancy options of subscribing to healthy meal plans, but most of us tend to find them monotonous and unaffordable in the long run. Again, my problem with the meal plans is that they are not customized as far as I know, and the portions can range from very little to too much, which we can't track. Nor can we understand the ingredients of the meals because 'healthy' is a very subjective term, and while a keto meal plan, which is heavy on the fats and avoids the carbs, works excellently for one person, someone else might face cholesterol fluctuations while having it on a daily basis.

You must also understand that your stomach is not a garbage can. Please refrain from loading up on the day's leftovers. I am the last person to advise you to throw your food away; I hate it when I see people doing this even at

public events or marriages. Nevertheless, please pay attention
to everything that you feed yourself and respect your body. If
you have a sizable portion of food left after your meal, make
a doggy bag and give it to someone else who needs it. If it is
a very small amount of leftover food, you could always feed it
to a stray or to your own pet, or put it in the refrigerator and
eat it a day or two later.

Eating right never starts off easy, but it becomes easier
when you start getting used to it.

Tips to Help You Get Started on Meal Prepping

1. Make a list of what you already have, and then plan what
   you need to buy.
2. Decide what to make. Start with planning one meal (e.g.,
   lunch) that you can carry to work for the entire week.
3. Go grocery shopping on the day you do your meal prep.
4. Prep your meal. You could make soups or curries, chop
   veggies for salads or make a stir-fry without the dressing.
5. Store it in the refrigerator or freezer if necessary.

16

Zzzzzzzzzzzz

It has been a few years since I introduced routines into my life and everyday activity. People who know me well know that I am an early riser and early sleeper. I wake up around 5:30 a.m. on most days, and sometimes even at 4:30 a.m., especially on the days when I have to play badminton with my friends or complete a quick training session in the gym before catching a flight or going to a morning shoot. Similarly, I start yawning from 8:30 p.m. onwards, and I usually go to sleep by 9:30 p.m.

I don't wake up this early to prove a point to myself or to the world. Nobody cares about when you wake up, what you do when or at what time you sleep, and as long as you are successful, the world is a kind place for you. Over the years, I just became accustomed to waking up early. I find that it gives me a comfortable amount of silent time with myself for my morning routine—before the texts, calls and other noise and distractions start to pour in. I feel like I can get a lot done in the morning. It makes for a peaceful and productive start to my entire day.

Once I wake up, I make my bed, brush my teeth, offer a prayer in gratitude in front of the deities I have in my room, and then drink hot coffee to fully wake up before stepping out to finish my training. While the coffee is brewing, I meditate quickly. Once I finish my 60 minutes of intense training of lifting weights with my friends (having friends who work with your schedule is such a blessing indeed), I return home to spend some time with my mom at the kitchen counter. Then I drink my protein shake and bathe, following which my productive day starts at around 8 a.m., with me all fresh and pumped up with the dopamine rushing in. This almost never changes. I am so used to it that even on Sundays I wake up early, and though I don't work out I keep finding something to engage with in the morning to make it productive for me.

On the flip side, being a morning person does hamper my social life. My day usually comes to an end by sunset, so if I step out of the house after 7 p.m., there needs to be a really good reason for it. My friends used to make fun of me by saying that the lockdown actually made zero difference to someone like me. I am a very homebound person, and if I don't have to leave for work or travel, I prefer being by myself at home.

When you are in the entertainment business, you don't have a specific time when it comes to work. You could be called for work at sunrise (where you have to wake up at 3 a.m. and be ready by 5:15 a.m. at the location with makeup!), or have a 9 a.m.–6 p.m. workday (which works the best for me), or be called for a night shoot (the one I dread the most— 2 p.m.–2 a.m. or 9 p.m.–6 a.m.). Sometimes, when there is a deadline and I am under extreme pressure, I even have to work continuously without breaks, sometimes combining these call sheets together—all hell would break loose but I would pretend I have superpowers and work with a smile on my face for the love I have for the job!

I remember the night shoots from my anchoring days. They would invariably end at 3–4 a.m., at least on the days when we filmed for reality shows. Being the sole anchor of the show, I had to be in the frame from start to end. That meant about 10–12 hours of standing in my high heels, with the harsh lights beating down on my face and tiring me out. When the filming with judges, special guests and participants was over, I envied them as everyone except for me would get to leave; I had to stay back to do the anchor links (the introduction to the show, the sponsor mentions, break links, the conclusion and fillers, etc.). This part required more focus, and I needed to look fresh because there were close-up shots and the audience's attention would be on me when the show finally aired. I managed to pull myself up each time at 2 a.m. or 3 a.m. for one of these shoots, and I'd beg and pray to God to hear the words 'pack up' being uttered. Once I heard them, I wouldn't waste even a single and I'd run out of the studio with my footwear in my hand because my feet would be too sore and swollen most of the times.

When I'd be in my caravan to change and pack my stuff to leave, all the other artistes and technicians who were part of the show would normally gather in another caravan. I used to try to sneak out and get into the car to return home, but I was often asked to join them for dinner. Since my hunger would be by this time at its peak, having skipped meals in between (I would survive on chai and biscuits throughout the shoot),

I would often accept that offer, quickly reach a spot with my cold salad (eating salads frequently from this place where the raw vegetables were imported and stored for long months at a time was what gave me a lot of gut issues, as I realized much later) and gobble it up while eavesdropping on the gossip about the shoot, nodding and smiling in between in response to the conversations happening around me. Almost everyone on the set would be active and energetic whereas I would be totally exhausted, and this used to make me wonder why I was the odd one out in the group. It was the start of my realization that maybe I am a morning lark and not a night owl, or that the others were accustomed to this routine while my body was still getting used to it. When I got back home, the newspaper and milk packets would be in my doorway, and I would pick them up and be let into the house as my dear mom or dad would have woken up by then. I'd remove my make-up, bathe and then hit the hay with a sense of satisfaction after a good day's (or rather, a good night's) work. It doesn't sound terrible so far, does it? Well, the tragic ending is coming up next.

I would sleep for under three hours on such days when I had night shoots. I wasn't sure why. It could have been because I was overwhelmed after witnessing a lot of emotions during the shoot (for example, people crying when they lose during a round and are eliminated, or people excited and happy when they win). The exposure to the whole crowd, the noise and the lights also made matters worse. It could also have been due to the fact that I never had a regular sleep schedule and kept switching it based on my work and travel. I used to extensively travel outside India to host events during this time, and adjusting to different time zones and finding a way to get a few hours of sleep amidst all of the travelling was difficult too. The consequences of my messy sleep routine reflected in my energy levels, mood fluctuations, my productivity in what I did on those days after I had woken up, my eating habits and definitely the way I looked and felt about things too. I had people asking me why my face was puffy and why I had such visible dark circles at a young age. I would constantly open the fridge and look for sweets and chocolates to give me a rush of energy, my body would feel the pain of exhaustion and it would take at least two days since that point for me to get back to my usual form. My cortisol levels were high because of the lack of adequate sleep, which affected my eating too. I suppose that the era we were in allowed me to play around with my sleep schedule more than the present age.

Currently, if there are any dates when I have night shoots for any film project, I mentally prepare myself for it and map things out. I plan out a proper routine for the night before the shoot and the night after the shoot. I carry my food with me during the shoots so that I neither feel heavy nor starved. I have completely stopped drinking chai during shoots, compared to the five or six cups that I used to have even a few years ago. I also treat the twenty-four-hour period of my shoot as more of a jet lag period. This means that I don't push myself to sleep after the shoot in the morning, but have a good porridge or smoothie for breakfast and run errands or do activities to keep myself engaged (without involving too much of thinking or physical activity) until it's evening, after which I have an early dinner and go to sleep. By this time, my body would be craving for the sleep that I had skipped by waking up early in the morning, so it helps me get back to my regular sleep cycle and function normally after 8–9 hours of uninterrupted sleep at night. I also limit my use of electronic devices, focus on eating lightly without skipping meals and do some deep breathing exercises a couple of times as part of ensuring I keep my sanity in check during the long night shoots.

Even my socializing skills have been bolstered over time. These days, I usually try and persuade my friends and colleagues to meet me for lunch or coffee rather than make an appointment for dinner. This is because my brain functions at its best until about 5 p.m., after which I truly sense a shift. In fact, I prefer a nice, quick breakfast–work meeting these days.

Having explained so much, though I am an early riser, it is not necessarily true that everyone should do the same. I have read several books that associate waking up early with a successful life—I beg to differ here, for I know a lot of successful people who work in the night since they are more comfortable with that as people won't call or email them late in the night. It is the same as why waking up early in the morning works best for me. I know a person who spends his day with his kids, puts them all to sleep and then starts at around midnight and works all the way till dawn. He found that to be the most comfortable routine during the pandemic. The trick is to find 'your best productive time' and capitalize on it for your work instead of drinking and partying, if your aim is to succeed in the career that you have chosen.

But have you wondered about the evolutionary reason why we are supposed to sleep in the night and wake up in the morning? Why young children (3–10 years old) and old people (60+ years old) mostly tend to be active in the morning?

The speculation is that back when we were living as hunters and gatherers, the night was considered to be dangerous because of the darkness.[1] Hence, humans would hide in the caves to sleep and stay away from wild animals, and use the light during dawn to get out and hunt, pick food and bring it back to their tribe. I have read articles that indicate that nobody would get up at night to even go and urinate, out of fear, and instead wait till the morning when they could hear the sounds and movements of other people before getting up from their resting spot.

Evolution has made us associate our waking hours with the morning and sleeping hours with the evening or night. It is when kids hit adolescence and then become adults that this dissipates, and their time of sleep starts to deviate. Of course, research in this area is never concrete, and these are ideas which may or may not be true.

Another idea that is often discussed about sleep is that our retinal sensitivity to light goes up at night, and that might hamper with our melatonin levels which promote sleep.[2] Light inhibits melatonin, so there are claims that exposure to light affects our mood, metabolism, reproduction and turnover rates of skin and hair cells. To really understand how true this is, if you feel constant fatigue for no reason, you could probably check to see and understand how much light you are exposed

---

[1] See https://www.psychologytoday.com/us/blog/personal-health-mastery/201708/what-hunter-gatherers-tell-us-about-natural-sleep-patterns.

[2] See https://www.ncbi.nlm.nih.gov/pmc/articles/PMC1855314/#:~:text=Levels%20of%20melatonin&text=The%20hormone%20secretion%20increases%20soon,role%20in%20its%20hormonal%20activity.

to, and how much sleep you are getting—this is because sleep is an important factor in restoring good moods and energy levels.

Most people have a good idea of whether they are a morning or night person, but there are quite a lot of variables involved to understand why each of us prefers to sleep in a certain way. The diet before we sleep, what our day was like physically and mentally, our energy levels and our exposure to light are all key factors in understanding our circadian rhythms (sleep–wake cycle). Apparently, this also shifts from time to time. There was a phase in my own life when I wouldn't sleep before 12:30 a.m. and couldn't wake up before 9 a.m. in the morning. I couldn't have imagined back then that I would become this person today!

As much as science is providing answers based on what works under specific, controlled conditions, the area of research is expanding by the day and so it can't address all the situations in which you or I live. There are truly a lot of variables that can impact sleep and wakefulness, and I assembled a few important tools below that you have control over and can use to probably experiment with without coming to any definite conclusions. This is just to make records and take note of how you are doing with these conditions. You don't even have to change the way you are handling your sleep now, but this was interesting for me to understand myself, so I have included it here for you to try out too:

1. Write down for each day when you went outside to get sunlight:
    E.g., 30th July

W: 6:15 a.m. SL: 7 a.m./4 p.m. D: 40 min
(W stands for wake-up time; SL stands for sunlight time;
D stands for how long the exposure to sunlight was)

2. Write down the time of your meals for each day:
    E.g., 30th July
    M: 8 a.m., 11 a.m., 2 p.m., 5 p.m., 8 p.m.
    (M stands for meals)

3. Write down when you exercised:
    E.g., 30th July
    Ex: 7 a.m. and 5 p.m.
    (Ex stands for exercise)

This is not to make you obsess over your sleep cycle, and I
don't suggest you do this for longer than a week. By doing
this, I found an interesting pattern about myself when it comes
to waking, light viewing and exercising, and that helped me
sense where I had my problems and how to fix them. For
example, on the days when I exercised early in the morning, I
felt that my sleep lasted longer than on days when I exercised
in the evenings (my body temperature was going up in the
latter half of the day). In fact, I even realized that taking a cold
shower in the evenings helped my quality of sleep improve
drastically. But this is just what happens to me; maybe things
will be different for you. Try this experiment carefully, without
being reckless about it. If you find it overwhelming to do all at
once, try doing just one thing at a time for a week.

    With all of that, I hope you have a good sleep today!

17

Sorry, I Don't Care

There are some typical comments that people make about others' bodies. For example, if you have put on a little weight, when they see you they will exclaim, 'Oh you have grown so fat!'

If you're underweight, they will surely say that you have grown 'too skinny'!

If you're of average build, they might offer a generic comment like 'You are neither this nor that'.

If you're dusky, you're 'too dark', and if you're light-skinned, you're 'too fair'.

If you have thick, long hair, it's 'old-fashioned', and if you have short hair, they might say that 'long hair suited you so much better'.

Dealing with similar opinions that other people have has been a struggle for me forever. From what I wear, to how much make-up there is on my face, everything gets dissected in an over the top manner day in and day out. I realized after several times of feeling broken, hurt and insecure that this is a never-ending and vicious cycle. Unless we as victims come to terms with this and seek a mechanism to get out of the cycle, it will drown us in the toxicity that it is made of.

Even during my time at school, I was someone who was trying too hard to get accepted into the popular groups. I remember the time when all my classmates were once talking about a certain pop song by Britney Spears, and I had never heard it nor did I have a clue about who Britney was back then. While they were having this conversation about the song and how sexy she looked in it, I was just nodding along and pretending as if I knew about it when I had zero idea about what they were saying, all to be a part of the conversation. Now when I look back to those days and moments, I just wish I was myself and admitted to not knowing what the song was all about. I am so passionate to write about this today because I wish someone had drilled this into my head while I was in school.

To all the people who have been or are in this same place that I am talking about, I just want to sum this up by saying that you don't have to do what your crowd wants you to do. Most of the time, if you backtrack to see when someone had picked up habits of smoking or drinking alcohol, it would have mostly started while in school or college, and would have begun due to peer pressure or to impress their group of friends. Doing anything in life for the sole purpose of pleasing people or getting into the good books of someone is just not worth it.

When I was doing well in the television industry, as much as I was happy and felt fulfilled about my work, I had to face the constant comparisons made between me and my other contemporary anchors, with media articles that argued about who was the best among all the anchors. They discussed questions like who was earning more and who had more fans and followers and so on. Though this made no difference in my work, I am sure that things would have been less awkward in my social relationships with those who were referred to in these articles. While I was trying to be the most passionate one in my job, the constant comparisons made me want to seek out being the best, which wasn't necessary at all.

Then there are the constant opinions about bodies that people have—not about their bodies, but that of others. These opinions only make us feel more terrible about our bodies, as if we have done something wrong. It is hard as it is for us to be able to accept our bodies for what they are. Even for me, as much as some of you might think that I am a health coach now and I know it all and crush my body goals easily, social media exposure does affect me too. I have my down days as well, even if they are fewer in number than before. There are days when I still feel gloomy, doubt my abilities and my body and compare it with the bodies of others as well. This is probably a good time to dissect this.

I normally use a calorie deficit or a 'mini cut' programme only when I need to look a specific way for work-related reasons, for it definitely takes a toll on my body. After I finish the 'mini cut' programme and get the results I want, I go back to my maintenance regime and recover my metabolism by eating more and working out less aggressively. Thus, my body naturally won't look as it did earlier when I was on the maintenance mode, and I'm fine with it when I need to do this for my own health reasons. But sometimes somebody would spot me and come say, 'Hey R, you were looking great 4 weeks ago. What happened now, it looks like you have gained some weight on your face!' and I simply wouldn't know what to say in response. This would negatively affect me quite regularly. I would just stop the maintenance programme wherever it was, and go back to the calorie restriction programme, thus attaching too much value to the comment made by people like these.

However, after a few times of this happening, I gave myself a talking to, and decided to filter out and discard these random comments that people would chuck at me. I started working on making the choice between self-sabotage and learning to brace up. Things like this won't ever stop until we decide to change our mindset. It was difficult to start with it, but now I feel really comfortable in my skin and I am able to handle such comments. When someone tells me that I have gained weight compared to my last Instagram post on a comment below the post, I just smile and ignore it; if they dare to mention it to my face, I usually tell them, 'Yeah, the point was to gain weight.'

Even now, no matter how many months or years later you are reading this book, if you go check my posts on Instagram, there will be a whole lot of comments talking about my body and the way I look, trying to put me down. There was someone who saw me two days ago when I was taking my dog on a walk. All he had to say to me was, 'Hi, sorry but you look so thin now. Please go back to being the "Bubbly Chubby Ramya"'. I just smiled and moved along. Recently, while I was scrolling through my messages on Instagram, I read a message from someone that said, 'You have a big face and small body.' I am not sure what comments like these imply, but I do wonder where people get this sense of entitlement from. Some think that I am really thin, whereas others think that I have put on weight! The other day, my friend reminded me of the time when two men rushed over to us on seeing us jogging at the beach, only to stop us and ask, 'How do you look so white?' (talking about my complexion). This obsession with complexion is also something that I don't understand. On several occasions even other women have walked up to me and pointed out that I look 'nice and fair' in person but 'dark' on television. What's wrong if I were darker? Why is it something that has to be pointed out? Some of my friends in school used to make fun of me by saying that I was fortunate to be fair-skinned, because if I had been wheatish or dark nobody would have given me a second look. This was supposed to be funny of course—you only need to look at our movies and TV shows in Tamil, where commenting on someone's clothes, their skin colour and their body seems to be the easiest way to crack people up. Even though we are in an age where we talk about body positivity, people still enjoy and find humour in making fun of others and their bodies.

For the longest time, I think I suppressed this want or need in me to feel sexy and desirable, at the expense of keeping up with the conservative, saree-clad image that I had of me. I felt like I had to live up to that image of someone who won't go against society's norms. That's why throughout my teens and early 20s, I never wore some of the dresses or shorts that I so badly wanted to sport, since the fear of being judged stopped me from buying them. I would just observe myself in the mirror in the trial rooms, and then leave without buying them. However, after I started powerlifting (more on this in the chapter on powerlifting) and I worked on making decisions just for myself, ignoring others and their opinions, I felt liberated. I feel like I started living my life to its fullest ever since. I truly believe that I can be a muscular, athletic and strong powerlifter, and yet someone who can be feminine too. You can look any way you want and still be able to wear the clothes that you want to wear confidently without seeking external validation. It is your body, after all. When I switched from wearing loose salwars and full-sleeve kurtis to draping my sarees with enhancing neckline blouses that were fitting and wearing dresses and tank tops and tights for workouts, I revamped my wardrobe and started buying clothes without overthinking things. They were no longer clothes that I simply bought left untouched, since I actually started wearing what I wanted to wear. It felt really good. It made me extremely confident and more expressive as a person too. My happiness was simply infectious. Though there was an initial resistance from a few detractors who had not seen me that way before, they gave up on offering any advice about my choice of clothes when they realized that their opinions made no difference to me.

Others' opinions about ourselves have to be taken with a pinch of salt. Sometimes they are well-intentioned, but at other times they are just flung at us to prick us. In our society, women are generally conditioned to value others' opinions more than their own. A big part of why women struggle so much in making their point or feeling valued is because we take these social norms, people's expectations and opinions and weaponize them against ourselves. Things won't change until every woman's mind changes on this matter. That is why

I feel it is important to reiterate this, as many times as it is required: your body belongs only to you!

You can decide not to lose the fat. You can decide to lose some fat and then discontinue the process. You can decide on some eating habits that you want to change or the specific goals that you want to achieve. If you decide to lose fat, you can decide how much of it you want to reduce. You can wear anything you want to wear, for your own sake. All of this is absolutely okay. Only you get to decide these things, and no one else has any right to tell you otherwise.

I have no interest in all of us looking the same, making the exact same choices and having the exact same lifestyles. My interest and passion are all about equipping women from all walks of life from all parts of the world with the right tools for them to overcome their struggles, particularly their weight and food struggles. That's my vision—to celebrate our bodies the way they are.

Making unapologetic decisions is a skill that helps in finding and creating true freedom and power about what you want for yourself, for your body and your relationship with food. It is not about making decisions based on what someone else will think. The decision comes from a powerful place. Over time, these help empower an individual and what they believe in. That is what we want to achieve—the empowerment of the individual so we can rebuff society's expectations or standards.

18

The Pros and Cons

I've always been the kind of person who analyses and overthinks every situation that comes my way. At times, this has helped me, but at other times, it has made things more complicated than necessary.

Since you are reading my book and we are exploring my thought patterns now, I'd like to introduce you to my world of pros and cons. Here are some of the pros and cons of working out:[1]

Pros

1. It increases your energy levels: While a lot of you might think that exercising will drain your energy and make you

---

[1] See- https://www.healthline.com/nutrition/10-benefits-of-exercise#TOC_TITLE_HDR_7. Also https://www.mayoclinic.org/healthy-lifestyle/fitness/in-depth/overuse-injury/art-20045875#:~:text=Common%20causes%20of%20overuse%20injury&text=An%20overuse%20injury%20typically%20stems,lead%20to%20an%20overuse%20injury and https://greatist.com/grow/when-exercise-makes-you-overeat#1.

tired, the very opposite of that is true. It will invigorate you and will allow you to do everything more enthusiastically.

2. It boosts your memory: If you're constantly forgetting your house keys, the route to a familiar destination, or dates and names, exercising will help keep your mind alert and will keep stress at bay, thus acting as a memory stimulant.

3. It gives you radiant skin: Day in and day out, people ask me what I do to maintain my skin, and I just keep saying that it's 'exercise'! This is the truth. Working out and sweating really help to flush out those toxins and release those endorphins. I feel pumped up after a workout session and it gives me what I like to call a 'gym glow'. So when you work out, you also get a complimentary facial!

4. It improves your sleep quality: Well, of course! A good workout intensely challenges every muscle in your body, so that by the end of the day, you crave that good eight–hour sleep. Even if you want to stay awake and party hard, you simply can't. And I think that's a good thing!

5. It keeps you young: When you get fit and sleep well, you will notice that you start to have supple skin. This glow up is the natural outcome. You start looking and feeling young, and signs of ageing reduce visibly.

Cons

1. It increases the chances of injury: If you're careless while training, have a trainer who misguides you or have no trainer at all while lifting heavy weights, it can result in serious injuries for life.

2. You'll become almost too disciplined: Have you noticed people sometimes excusing themselves from a house party you're hosting or calling it a night at around 9 p.m.? They probably follow a clockwork regime of waking up early and finishing their morning exercises before the rest of the day takes over. They do not want to compromise on their routines. As much as this is a great habit (I myself am a classic example of this), if you're someone who enjoys eating out and partying every few days, this is not something you can easily balance. You can't have both in this case, and need to make your choice.

3. Your family might perceive you differently: Our women have always been told to put others before themselves and to make sacrifices for the family. When you suddenly switch your focus to your body, your nutrition intake and your workout regime, your family might perceive you as being selfish if they haven't seen it before.

4. It will make you devour food: Exercise helps increase your appetite, but you have a choice between eating smart and healthy after a workout and wolfing down your next meal. I have seen people extensively exercising—two hours of cycling, three hours of badminton, ninety minutes of walking—only to stop at the very popular Sangeetha or Saravana Bhavan restaurants straight afterwards, and gorge on sambar, *vadai*, pongal and filter *kaapi* each time. This is only going to make all your efforts go down the drain. Following an exercise routine is meant to complement your process of fat loss—the thought that you can eat absolutely anything because you've finished working out is a fallacy.

Therefore, I'd say that you should weigh the pros and cons and decide on what you'd like to do.

According to me, everybody should exercise in some way and choose an activity that they enjoy, so that they can be disciplined at it. We're no longer in the Stone Age where our work involves regular physical activity by default. Having said that, please consult your physician and check on your dos and don'ts before starting out.

To people who feel 'exercise and dieting' are too expensive for their way of living, please erase from your mind the wrong notion that you need to spend a lot of money to stay healthy. All you need is a good understanding of nutrition and of your body.

If spending money on a high-end gym and personal trainer is too expensive, joining boot camps and group sessions can be a more economical form of exercising that can be opted for.

Even going for a walk every day, skipping, playing an outdoor game and learning a recreational activity are simple forms of exercise that can help you steadily increase your physical activity.

Choose what works for you and keeps you motivated . . . and don't forget to keep on moving!

Now that we have the basics covered, let's go a few steps further . . .

Part III

Fitness Myths and Methods

19

My Relationship with Food

Like everyone else, my relationship with food has changed with time. In fact, I notice that it never stays fixed anymore. There isn't a rule book that I follow, or strict eating times and fixed habits that I stick with.

As you know from the previous chapters, I did not suddenly decide to change my eating patterns one day. It is a matter of experience and being aware of my relationship with food. I would say that this has been a process of learning from the bad choices I have made when it comes to eating. If you feel that the things I am mentioning here are too unrealistic, you need to know that your relationship with food is not something that can be fixed magically, but it is a process that needs to be worked on consistently. Much like my past and present situations are not comparable, you shouldn't compare your achievements with mine. Our experiences will naturally differ.

To give you some perspective about my changing relationship with food, the earlier chapters were mostly about how food habits affected me while I was growing up. Some of my earliest memories were of watching my brother pick his racket to go play tennis while I was made to learn dance and music, which has been the case for most South Indian homes until recently. Women learning a sport or going to train in the gym from a young age had not been normalized. I am so happy to see the change now, and I secretly envy the women who have this privilege now. I strongly believe that it is easier to manage getting strong, being healthy and staying fit if you start at a young age.

As a child, I was not prohibited from eating anything. My parents never said no to ice cream, samosa, French fries or pizza. There was a phase when I only ate butter naan with paneer butter masala and vegetable biriyani from fast food joints every day for about two months. My parents put up with all the things I did even when I was in my extreme diet phase. I used to just eat raw salads for lunch, and even when we travelled to the remotest of villages and towns for pilgrimages deep in the South, my mom would find that one place which would cut vegetables and add some salt or pepper and give it to me for I would skip the meal and starve otherwise. I am glad I have changed for the better now.

Thus, my experiences with food in childhood and adolescence were not great to begin with. Like I mentioned before, I was not forbidden from eating anything, and there were a lot of treats available for me at any given point. When I went to college, I was constantly trying to lose weight. Because of what I'd read and heard and seen, I tried out what most others end up doing—I cut down on all the foods that I loved, the foods that were 'unhealthy'. This is what led to a constant binge and restrict cycle. I would do really well from Monday to Thursday, but when Friday came, I would lose control and eat all the foods that were 'restricted', which included pizza, ice creams, cookies, chips and so on. Following that, I would feel guilty, and by Monday I would tell myself the same thing again: 'Okay, this time, I will buckle up. This time, I'm going to focus and do better'. After several failed attempts over the years, I have learnt that this cycle never works. If you are in the same place now and this resonates with you, I want to emphasize that this method did not work for me. This is not sustainable, and I could not keep up with this cycle for a long time.

After all the diets, starvation, fasting and the wavering that I did, it wasn't until I learned about and started doing macro counting that I lost the weight that I had been trying to lose for a decade. Macro counting was not only effective, but also a fun and enjoyable way to achieve my goals. It allowed me to find that balance. I will tell you how to get started with this in an exclusive chapter.

That is enough about my history with food. Let us move on to my current relationship with food.

The first thing I want you to know is that I don't track unnecessarily anymore. I had started my fitness journey as a powerlifter who ate and used all the food primarily to prepare for lifting and during the competitions that I participated in. Once I felt like I needed a break there, I started to track macros for a couple of years for some very specific goals, like having a flat stomach. I had to go on a calorie deficit diet and track my food every day and log it to be able to gradually reduce my body fat percentage and get to the point of seeing visible changes in the abdominal area.

Since then, I haven't had any specific goals, and I am content with my strength and muscle mass too. I don't want to be excessively lean, and I am simply enjoying my High-Intensity Interval Training (HIIT) and strength workouts. I am at a maintenance phase when it comes to eating as well. I understand my nutrition, my body's needs and my portions too from all the years of tracking.

This doesn't mean that I am sitting and mentally calculating all the macros nowadays.

What works for me is being aware of the food that I eat during the day, and when it is time to eat lunch or have a snack, I just ask myself what I am deficient in for that day. This helps me understand what I need to improve on for my next meals. For example, if I have a lot of carbs for breakfast (*pesarattu*, idli) and lunch (rice, chapatti), I try to keep to focus more on protein for dinner (eggs, tofu and veggies or protein shakes). So, I generally track my macros mentally to balance them out evenly, and I do pay specific attention to my protein intake with the appropriate food selections in every meal to ensure I hit my protein goal by the end of the day.

Tracking macros for a period of time helps one understand portion sizes and the nutritional composition of food. For example, when I see a banana I know that I will mostly receive carbs from it, when I see tofu I know it'll mostly be protein and so on. The best thing is that this information never leaves your brain once you have tracked for a considerable period of time, and this helps you make choices even afterwards, once you have stopped tracking.

The second thing I want you to know is that I never feel guilty about any of my food choices.

I know you might be thinking, 'It's easy enough for you to say that because you are probably always eating healthy'. But that is not true. I too chose to indulge myself a few times. I stick to the 80/20 rule, where 20 per cent of my food choices will be something that won't be tagged as 'healthy'. Honestly, I have also started seeing food from a scientific angle, and there is no emotion or shame that I associate with food and food choices anymore. I have not always been this way. There have been times when I have eaten too much at one go, making me feel terrible about it later on. But this shift in attitude is because I have learnt and emerged from what used to drag me down before.

The next thing to know is that I love food and I overeat food.

Are you not able to believe me on that one? Let me elaborate.

There is a difference between binging on food and overeating.

Overeating is eating past satiety to a point where your stomach hurts or you don't feel good about the amount of food that you have eaten.

Binging is not a choice that you make, but rather something that happens to your body where you eat without thinking.

My close friends have seen me overeat several times. A few months ago, when one of my friends, who is a home baker, made a terrific chocolate caramel cake, I shamelessly had about half of the 1 kg cake all by myself. My friends were all shocked at watching me eat so much in one go, since this is a rare sight for them too. I had eaten too much to feel good about it. Later that night, and on the next day, I felt heaviness and discomfort in my stomach—it was such a bad experience for me. I have to reiterate that I did not feel any shame or guilt. I just told myself that I would be more careful the next time.

What I want to convey is that being healthy doesn't have to be about restricting all the foods you enjoy and eat to consume bland and oil-free food all the time. Even I choose to overeat at times, and live life without any limitations placed on what I eat.

The other thing is that I don't always align my food choices with my goals.

Every single thing I do need not be aligned with a goal or with a certain outcome. Living life with constant calculations is not the point.

To be cognizant of my choices is the primary goal that I pursue. Sometimes, I may make a short-term choice (for enjoyment) over a long-term benefit (a big goal)—that is still preferable to me since it is a conscious choice.

Unlike me, some of you might be thinking that you do not make these short-term choices and you aren't usually able to control what you do. This is where I come in as a coach to help you work on it.

Consistency is very important to get the results you want.

There is always this balance between the results that I want and what I'm willing to give up for it, and being honest with myself and understanding how to develop my mindset to achieve that goal is where everything begins. If I don't understand the process I am beginning, I will not be able to get the results I want. Getting this clarity greatly helps me, no matter what my goal is. If I'm on a certain regime and my birthday comes in between, I would work my way around eating a birthday cake and not worrying about tracking for that time period. But I do understand that when I make these choices, they will impact my results. Being aware of the consequences helps me make the choice with a clear conscience. However, if I am particularly determined at a point in time, where it is more important to see the results I want, then neither birthday dinners nor cakes can really stop me from getting distracted while I'm on that regime.

One thing I often hear from my clients is about spontaneous food, i.e., the food that is suddenly given at a friend's home, the food that is bought in the store for the kids at home, etc. In such situations, I encourage them to pick based on their circumstances and the type of food that is being offered. However, if it includes some food that you particularly struggle with, politely and firmly refuse to eat it.

Lastly, I never tell myself that I cannot eat something.

I never struggle when it comes to choosing to eat.

When you see a certain food, one half of you might want to give in to temptation while the other half might constantly remind you of your aim to lose fat. This dilemma doesn't feel good. Both of these parts belong to you, and if one wins, the other loses.

Restriction happens only when you tell yourself that you cannot have something. I no longer have any exceptions like 'cheat days', 'treats', 'rewards' or 'celebrations' when it comes to what I eat, since I know that I can eat anything anytime I want. This is what works for me, and it might work for you as well!

Let's discuss a few tangible examples to get the hang of the difference between what is a choice and what is a restriction.

I am a big fan of *basundhi* (a sweet similar to ras malai), whereas one of my cousins dislikes it completely. Let's say we go to a function where it is served, and if I see it and say, 'Oh my god, this looks delicious . . . too bad I can't have it, as I'll gain weight'—that would be a restriction.

But for my cousin, that cup of *basundhi* would not be enticing, exciting or something he might want to have even if it was offered to him. This is his choice here.

So, we both choose not to have the cup of *basundhi*, but our thoughts and feelings which lead to our decisions on this matter are entirely different.

The point I am making is that you can choose to have whatever it is that you want—nobody should tell you otherwise. If you choose to not eat something, that choice must be voluntary rather than motivated by external reasons or any restrictions. This is a fine line to tread, and an important point to understand.

Thus, I don't believe that there is a right way and a wrong way to have a relationship with food. I just wanted to provide my perspective on food and the relationship I have with it in this chapter so that you can think about your own food choices. If things aren't going too well for you currently, try out some of the methods that have worked for me. We should stop asking questions like 'Is this the right way to eat?' or 'Am I doing it correctly?' and start asking questions like 'Is this effective for me?' and 'Is what I am doing going to lead me to my long-term goals?'.

I didn't have all this guidance right from childhood. But I am glad that I at least learnt about this and adapted to it after becoming an adult. You can be the one who breaks that chain and make that change for your children or grandchildren.

Go for it!

20

'I Don't Eat Much but
I Can't Lose the Fat'

This was a common statement I'd make to every dietician and trainer in the early days of my fitness journey. Every time I said this, they would tell me that I was probably not consuming the right amount of food because I was guessing the portions I was supposed to eat. This was true in my case. We never know how much we are actually eating in terms of the portions, nor are we aware of the density of calories and nutrients in the food we eat until and unless we start tracking them or take expert help to calculate what is needed for our body and are given a chart to follow. The truth is, one can't possibly consume thin air and still not lose weight.

But it is not just that. When I started on a targeted fat loss goal, the initial 6–7 kg and inches were pretty easy and straightforward to lose. I just had to be disciplined and consistent with my training and eating—that's all it took to see the results. But the closer I came to my final goal and the lesser fat I had to lose from my body, the harder it became to achieve. The weight on the scales just stopped moving, I was increasingly demotivated and frustrated, and everything was going south.

This was the point when I realized that having 'cheat meals' once a week isn't all that great, because the real difficulty was when I went out in the weekend with my family to eat. Irrespective of whether I chose to eat something healthy or indulged myself a bit, my weight would immediately spike up for the next 3–4 days, and then return to where it was before. I used to feel like I was stuck in this cycle fluctuating weight, and ultimately making no progress.

The first thing I learnt was to stop obsessing over the number on the scale. I realized that the best thing to do is to average out the measurement every ten days. Then I could take that into consideration as my actual progress, instead of feeling frustrated at the scale which added up my water retention, salt intake, bloating because of food that I ate outside, the fibre and roughage bulk that was adding extra weight, my hormonal fluctuations and so on.

Let me state the difference between fat loss and weight loss as I know it:

We are all very familiar with weight loss and we always use this term when talking about wanting to size down. When I began this journey, I was more familiar with weight loss than fat loss. If I stand on the scale and the scale goes up, that means I have gained weight, and if it goes down it means that I have lost weight.

I would often freak out when the scale went up, for that meant to me that I had gained 'fat', which led to gaining weight as well. Now I know that it is much more complicated than this because our weight in general corresponds to much more than just the fat in our body. We have muscles, soft tissue, organ weight, water weight and ligaments, all of which correspond to the weight we see on the scale. These can fluctuate based on various situations, including our hormonal imbalances, salt in the diet, the liquids we consume and so on. That is why when we see the scale go up or down by a kilogram, we cannot necessarily equate that to fat gain or loss.

I realized that I could lose fat without losing any weight. Conversely, I can also lose weight without losing any fat! This is the concept that is often misunderstood, and the next time you want to say that you want to lose weight, you should instead rephrase it by saying that you want to lose fat since that is probably what you mean (why would you want to lose water, tissues and muscles anyway?).

To lose fat, we need to create a calorie deficit (eat fewer calories than you burn). That is it. End of story. So another shift of thought that is required here is that whatever it is that you believe is working for you or for someone you know (in terms of a certain kind of diet regime) is not the diet by itself, but the calorie deficit it creates that causes the fat loss. This can happen through restricting their eating window and thus reducing the overall calorie intake—if it's Intermittent Fasting (IF)—or removing a macro nutrient which is going to reduce the calories (keto or paleo diet) and so on. No matter what diet you opt to do, this is the basic idea behind it. Therefore, if you eat above your calorie deficit on a ketogenic diet or on IF, you still won't lose the fat.

Coming back to the basics of not simply guessing the portions of your food, understanding the portions of what I eat and weighing them on a food scale was a game changer. Weighing my food actually did clean up the 100 calories here and 150 calories there that I was eating without realizing. I did not stop eating outside once a week, because I needed to do that to maintain a sense of normalcy and not be deprived of anything, but at the same time, I didn't stop logging the food I ate outside either. This way, I knew how many calories I had overshot when I was eating out, and I would balance that out on the next two days by adjusting my calories accordingly and paying closer attention to eating even more vegetables to keep me full. For example, if my calorie deficit was 1450, instead of eating 1450 calories all day, I was playing around with it to give me better freedom. The average of 1450 multiplied by 7, i.e., 10,150 calories was what mattered to me, and this was my calorie budget. So, if I had a high calorie day of 1700 on a day when I went out, on the next two days I would have low calorie days of 1300 to balance things out. Ultimately, when I take all the days and add them together and divide by 7, my average would come to 1450.[1]

The other perspective I understood here is that as my weight and my body fat percentage reduced, so would my maintenance calories (this was information I had gathered from my trainer). This is because metabolically I had a new body by this point. That is part of the reason why the old calorie range won't work at times for some people after a while. So the macros and calories keep changing, and they need to be shifted based on this change that we see in the body every few

---

[1] https://www.healthyway.com/content/the-big-picture-a-weekly-calorie-allowance/.

months. This information above may seem easy to follow and clear but I assure you that unless you start this with expert guidance and information, this will not work the way you want it to and lead to unnecessary health problems.

When we think about fat loss, what I realized with all of this is that it can't be reduced to a few steps that are copied and precisely followed. You need to be in a deficit for a while and then get to the maintenance phase when things slow down, and again cycle back to the deficit to see effective results. When this became clear to me, I started anticipating fluctuations in my weight while on the maintenance phase because it was totally normal. To put it logically, the weight I had initially lost was nothing but the water weight, so I knew that what was coming back during maintenance was the same water weight. The mistake is when most people, especially women who fear weight gain, doubt the process when there is an initial increase in weight, and pull back from the method altogether.

In a normal scenario, anyone who starts on a diet or an activity that helps them lose body fat will see their results initially, because the body will suddenly find that it is being given less food than normal or made to burn more calories than what it usually does. This is why I was seeing initial benefits when I had started as well. But over the course of time, when we keep eating less than usual, the body understands that this is the new normal and adapts to the change. At the end of the day, our bodies don't care about aesthetics, and its job is to protect us by storing as much fat as possible to be prepared for a time when we might not give it external food (for instance, when we are in danger). So, by eating less (calorie deficit) for long periods of time, we suppress our metabolism. Most women undereat with the fear that eating even a bit more than usual will make them gain weight, thus making this calorie deficit their maintenance calories! Do you see where this is going wrong? I was doing exactly this for the longest time too! I used to think, what if I become fat? What if my clothes don't fit me? What if I look fluffy and unfit on camera? These were the constant questions that pulled me away from trying to increase my calorie intake.

This idea that we have never truly changes unless we give a chance for our body to restore our metabolism. As you know now, with undereating or starving, your body will eventually adapt (metabolic adaptation) and learn to survive within the new limits, so you won't continue to lose weight like you did at first. We call this a 'fat loss plateau'. Although this can be reversed by slowly and consciously eating more in a planned and distributed way, it isn't easy to do this, and you need to be really patient during the process to set it back. What would need to be done in such a case is to first calculate your maintenance calories (the calories that your body requires in totality for maintaining your ideal weight typically), which by this time will be much higher than what you are intaking currently, and then you achieve the requirement by building your calories slowly from your current deficit or jump into maintenance in one go—once you complete your fat loss phase. I normally do it slowly by adding 100 calories or so per week from my last calorie deficit until I get to my maintenance phase and then stay at that for 2–3 months at least.[2] If done

---

[2] https://aaptiv.com/magazine/reverse-dieting.

with the right guidance, you won't gain any fat nor much weight in the process (if that is your concern—and that is mostly the concern for most of my female clients), and it will rather make you happy as now you will get to eat more food that you enjoy. Additionally, your body will get to use the energy to push harder during your workouts, which means you will get more definition and muscle too. Of course, bear in mind that you might take a few weeks or months to repair your metabolism, depending on how long you have made your body feel deprived of food. This is a project that you must not be in a rush to finish.

This is why I understand what professional bodybuilders or bikini models undertake—since their lives are about looking a certain way for their survival, they tend to keep shifting their calorie intake from time to time. They aggressively eat less during their prep time for a given competition and consume higher calories after competing to use that to recover and build their metabolism. This is ideally what I do too, depending on my requirements,

So, this is the glitch in the system that often goes unnoticed when you are on a fat loss journey and you stop seeing results over time. It's really important to figure out what is going wrong and tweak it. What I myself do these days when I am on a cutting diet is to go to my calendar and mark out six weeks as my deficit window. Then I'll know that my goal for the next six weeks is to hit my calorie deficit of whatever I calculate (I will be sharing this in the chapter about macros). But after the six weeks is over, I will go back to eating my maintenance calories and not continue the calorie deficit, whether or not I have attained my goal. Will the scale go up? Yes. But is that acceptable? Of course, it is. I always get very excited when I get to the maintenance phase because it is like having a surplus in your budget to shop for whatever you want. For me, this is also the real challenge—to be smart about whatever else I eat and strike a balance.

This maintenance phase actually works out differently for each of us, and what can influence things here is what we choose to eat while we're in this phase. The extra calories can be substituted with more processed food or healthy options. I have seen that there is hardly any difference when I choose to eat in maintenance compared to when I am on a calorie deficit, except that I eat more portions to add the hundreds of calories in each meal for maintenance. I found that this made my body stronger, I looked healthier and defined and I felt more energetic. However, when the foods I chose during the maintenance phase were more like indulgences or snacks, I found myself to be hungrier, more lethargic and looking more bloated than usual. I showed greater weight fluctuations as well. Don't get me wrong here—I am someone who can't go without indulgences and won't ever deprive my clients or myself from treats entirely, but after I made this mistake the first time during maintenance, of spending all the extra calories on junk food, I learnt my lesson. It is better to increase the calorie allowance the times when I indulge occasionally than spend the extra calories I get while on maintenance every day on treats. So the more consistent I am with my eating behaviour during the maintenance phase, the lesser fluctuations I see on the scale. The other thing is that that I still need to make it my mission to weigh in all the food that I eat and note them down. It's like I become a scientist and conduct these little experiments to become more aware of my body.

The maintenance phase lasts as long as I want it to, and until I feel ready to go back to the calorie deficit, but I give it a minimum of at least two weeks, especially if I was in a plateau. I guarantee that when this is done the way I have mentioned, you will definitely start seeing those changes which were too stubborn to appear earlier.

I think that we as humans tend to become sloppy over time in what we do, whether we have to learn a new skill, apply for a new job or start studying a new course. It is not the end of the world, since that's how we are wired to behave. This is true for the calorie deficit journey as well, and the trick with the maintenance phase is that it fixes what was going wrong while we were doing the deficit. It's totally worth it. It works each and every time for me.

Now, if you are thinking about how I became such a geek, it was my interest in the subject. It made me read, talk to experts and try out the methods myself to see if they worked. During our journey towards the health goal, it is the action plan, and especially sticking to the plan, which makes all the difference in the world. Also, please take maintenance breaks. Practice it, get some expert help if you need to and do it responsibly. The more you do maintenance, the better it is for you. And to all of you who get worried about their metabolism, this is the one thing that you can do to fix it. Downgrading your calories over and over and eventually making that your maintenance will not help in the long term.

21

My Name Is Calories and
I Am Not Your Enemy

We find the word calories commonly used across all supermarket items, our smart watches and even on treadmills. We use them in discussions on food, tracking calories and identifying how many calories we burn from any physical activity.

What are calories?

A calorie is a unit of measurement that is used to identify how much energy we are putting into our body and how much energy the body is using.[1]

Basal Metabolic Rate (BMR), Total Daily Energy Expenditure (TDEE), Calorie Deficit and Calorie Surplus are other terms that we need to know while covering the topic of calories.

---

[1] https://www.nhlbi.nih.gov/health/educational/wecan/healthy-weight-basics/balance.htm#:~:text=What%20is%20Energy%20Balance%3F,physical%20activity%20is%20ENERGY%20OUT.

BMR is the amount of calories we need for our survival. Here, I am referring to the calories we burn while we rest. This includes the calories that are used by the body to function, such as by our heart to pump blood, lungs to fill up the oxygen, blood circulation, temperature regulation and so on and so forth.[2]

If you are curious to find out your BMR, one of the easiest ways to do it is to use an online calculator from the range of BMR calculators available now. For your convenience I am mentioning one such calculator for you here: www.calculator.net/bmr-calculator.html.

TDEE is the number of calories you burn in total, including from your physical activity. This not only refers to workouts but also to other movements such as walking around, working in the kitchen, doing a presentation in your office, chasing your kids while playing with them, etc. Your maintenance calories are the same as your TDEE.[3]

Calorie Deficit is when you are consuming fewer calories than your maintenance calories.

Calorie Surplus is when you are consuming more calories than your maintenance calories.

Let's assume person A burns 2400 calories per day to maintain his weight. When he reduces his intake of calories from anywhere between 1900–2100 calories per day and is on a deficit for a certain period of time, he will start losing fat. But at the same time, if there is a person B whose calories for maintenance is 1900, this would not help him lose the fat but

---

[2] https://www.healthline.com/health/what-is-basal-metabolic-rate.

[3] https://lifesum.com/nutrition-explained/calorie-maintenance-what-it-is-and-why-it-matters.

only help him to stay in the maintenance phase. For someone like me, I know that my current maintenance is roughly 1600 calories, and eating more than 2000 calories will be a calorie surplus and make me gain fat or muscle.

Note that I mentioned 'current maintenance' while referring to me. This is because as someone loses fat, the maintenance calories will also start lowering based on the lost fat. So, if I had started my tracking while I weighed 60 kg and in a period of six weeks I reached 54 kg, it's important for me to re-evaluate and understand my current maintenance. But that doesn't mean you keep eating lesser and lesser as your weight drops down too. Remember the earlier chapter about weight plateau and metabolic adaptations? This is why you need to keep changing things around a bit, and that's why I completely believe in the right mentoring and expert guidance when it comes to setting our goals for our health.

Are all calories the same?

Yes, they are, if this is only about calories as a number that we count to track.[4]

Also, calories are calories no matter when you consume them! But remember that while the calories in the food that you eat before 6 p.m. will be exactly the same after 6 p.m. as well, factors such as when you eat and what you eat matters in the long run for your metabolic improvements, digestion, sleep and hormone regulation. Practices such as having a balanced high-protein breakfast and a lean and light dinner

---

[4] https://www.runnersworld.com/beginner/a20809220/calorie-count-not-all-calories-are-created-equal/; https://millennialhawk.com/does-calorie-deficit-work-with-unhealthy-food/; https://www.insider.com/do-junk-food-diets-work-2017-6.

provide healthy payoffs in the long run beyond a weight loss goal.[5]

Your body sees food not as good or bad but considers merely its calories and macronutrient value, i.e., protein, fats and carbohydrates. While some food is nutrient dense, has higher calories and still won't keep you feeling full for long, others seen as 'healthy foods' tend to be advantageous for fat loss because they are more voluminous per kcal, more filling and more micro dense. For example, I can plan a 1600 kcal diet for a day with (2 pieces of) poori and potato masala, a can of cola, (2 slices of) cheesy pizza and a piece of cake and be done vs consuming tons of vegetables, soups, salads, fruits, lean proteins and whole foods to achieve the same amount of calorie intake. Though both would give me results from a weight loss perspective, trying to eat 1600 kcal of processed foods (as in the first example) will more likely result in far less filling, less voluminous food and which means that I will feel sluggish, bloated and very hungry. It won't be sustainable and will almost certainly lead to overconsumption or make me go off track in no time. Depriving yourself of all the foods you like and force feeding yourself broccoli and spinach will also make you get sick of dieting and give up entirely. Hence the concept of finding the balance. This means that swapping in a few pieces of chocolate (for 200 kcal) for of a serving of yoghurt and fruit one day will have zero effect on your weight loss goal, except that you may be slightly hungrier but slightly happier with the chocolate!

---

[5] https://www.nbcnews.com/better/pop-culture/meal-timing-weight-loss-does-it-matter-when-you-eat-ncna907091.

Whether you do intermittent fasting and skip your dinner, or whether you have only one meal a day after 6 p.m., at the end of the day you are simply making a choice to either consume or not consume calories if you merely look at calories from a physiological perspective.

There are people who have a very dogmatic approach and say that nothing apart from calories matter. While I partly agree with this like how I began on this topic, I strongly feel that the quality of your food also absolutely matters for your physical, mental and emotional health and that is where all calories are not the same too!

The calories in vs calories out model may work out for weight loss briefly but be mindful that the source of your calories is as important, if not more.[6] When I constantly swap that 75 kcal with 2 tbsp of Belgian chocolate ice cream ice cream (25g) over ½ a kg of greens, it will lead to a failure soon in not only keeping with the programme, but also affect my appetite, energy level and long-term health! Eating processed foods everyday even if it is not too much can pose a risk to medical conditions such as a leaky gut, autoimmune syndrome, inflammations, decreased insulin sensitivity and early type 2 diabetes, PCOD, thyroid-related issues and so on.[7]

Thus, it is not the calories but the composition of the nutrients in our food which makes all the difference.

---

[6] https://www.healthline.com/nutrition/calories-in-calories-out#beyond-the-model%E2%80%99.

[7] https://www.eatthis.com/junk-food-side-effects/.

Carbohydrates, fats and proteins are the three macronutrients (macros) which give nutrition to our body:[8]

1. Carbohydrate: 1 g = 4 cal

If you eat carbohydrate-rich food like rice, which is 90 per cent carbs: 25 g of raw rice = 100 calories

2. Protein: 1 g = 4 cal

If you eat protein-rich food like egg white, which is 80 per cent protein: 25 g of egg whites = 100 calories

3. Fat: 1 g = 9 cal

If you eat fat-rich food like cheese, which is 80 per cent fat: 25 g of cheese = 225 calories

Also, bear in mind that any alcohol = 7 calories per gram, and it is made up of sugar and starch that has absolutely no nutritional value.

Ultra-processed foods such as breads, cereals, desserts, soft drinks, biscuits and fried food often have high amounts of sugar, salt and fat. They are loaded with calories and we love them a lot, but the sad news is that they have absolutely no

---

[8] Nutritional values given here may not necessarily be accurate. Nutritional calculators are disparate in the way they reach numbers and the brand of a product and the way it is processed can radically change the nutritional value of any given food. The reader is advised to make calculations based on the ingredients they personally use, using their own preferred method, or consulting with a licensed nutritional expert.

nutrients that serve any purpose to our body internally, except for maybe giving us the joy of having them.

If you ask me why we don't feel full with these foods that we enjoy the most despite them being rich in calories, it is because they have very less thermogenic effect, water content and hence, less satiation and satisfaction.

Thermogenic effect or the Thermic Effect of Food (TEF) is the number of calories needed by our bodies to digest, absorb and process the nutrients from what we eat.[9]

Of all the foods we eat, protein has the highest thermogenic effect, followed by carbs and finally fats.

This is why processed foods that are high in fats and carbs (plus a whole lot of preservatives and additives) don't make us feel full and make us consume more and more of them.[10] We also don't feel great after having them normally, as opposed to having a meal with fresh foods, because technically we have eaten a lot of dense calories but biologically they have no value. They just make us feel heavy, groggy and sluggish.

While we think fruits are good for us, which they are, drinking fruit juice will shoot up the calories while taking off the pulp (fibre) that is the best part of the fruit. Liquids like water and green tea have low calories or none at all. Soft

---

[9] https://examine.com/topics/thermic-effect-of-food/; https://www.verywellfit.com/thermic-effect-of-food-1231350#toc-what-is-the-thermic-effect-of-food

[10] https://www.healthline.com/nutrition/junk-food-and-metabolism#TOC_TITLE_HDR_3; https://www.revolution-pts.com/blog/understanding-the-thermic-effect-of-food#:~:text=The%20energy%20required%20to%20digest,the%20energy%20provided%20by%20it.&text=So%20that%20means%20protein%20tops,used%20for%20digestion%20and%20metabolism.

drinks or a can of your favourite beverage can have 150 to 300 calories, depending on the brand you choose, and they have nothing but a huge amount of empty sugar that has zero nutrients and gives you a rush of energy spikes through insulin, which often goes unutilized and stored as fat by the body.

Knowing things like this is why I like to understand the caloric value of foods. In general, certain fruits, non-starchy vegetables, lean meats and poultry will have lower calories and energy in them, and that is why healthier people eat a lot to make up for the energy they need. High energy foods, like processed foods, pasta, pizza, fries, burger, noodles, desserts, rice, etc. will have a higher number of calories, and although you would want to consume less of these, chances are you will still not feel full and want to eat more of them, thereby eating a surplus of calories (excess energy) which get stored as body fat.

I am informing you all about this so that you can make some educated decisions, if and when you want to, for keeping fit and staying healthy.

My approach is not to make you become overtly conscious or obsessive about the calories you eat for every single thing you put into your mouth. For one final time, I want to make it very clear that I do not think it is sustainable for someone to live their life entirely without ever allowing an indulgence. That feels like prison to me—the 80/20 approach is ideal for me and enables me to eat healthy most of the time while not restricting myself entirely from anything that I might want to eat. What do I mean by 80/20? Let's discuss that in the next chapter.

22

The 80/20 Rule

80/20 is the new 50/50.

Take the case of relationships. I've realized that couples who invest 80 per cent of their time in each other while reserving a 20 per cent window of time for themselves have the most balanced relationships.

The same applies to money management. If you spend 80 per cent of your salary every month, but set aside 20 per cent for savings and investments, you'll be able to plan wisely for the future. It's a winning formula.

Fun fact: The 80/20 rule is also known as the Pareto Principle, which says that 80 per cent of outcomes come from 20 per cent of our inputs. The rule also suggests that we do more instead of doing less. At work, for instance, focusing on our most important tasks for the day leads to higher productivity, as opposed to spending hours on doing a bunch of smaller, lower-priority tasks.

I've applied the 80/20 rule to fitness too: 80 per cent of fat loss is linked to the food that you eat, while 20 per cent is linked to your physical activity. If this combination is worked on effectively, you will definitely start losing fat and also work your way towards a healthy lifestyle.

I've adapted this same rule to the idea of nutrition as well. For me, eating 80 per cent healthy every day, and giving myself 20 per cent allowance to indulge on treats has personally been the game changer. I realized that when you impose extremely strict restrictions on your eating, it gets really hard to sustain them. You begin to feel like you're being punished for wanting to get healthy. Another problem is that reserving all our cravings for a single meal at the end of the week rarely ever works in our favour, since we're most likely to go all out on that particular meal or day, thus spoiling the good outcomes of the entire week. Have you wondered whom we are cheating when we call it a 'cheat meal'? So yes, the 80/20 rule is my strategy and I believe in it. You should similarly figure out a strategy that works for you too or take help from an authorized nutritionist to find one.

Our eating patterns should never feel like a painful sacrifice but should be something we can sustain and enjoy. So, when we start eating 80 per cent right every day—real foods like veggies, nuts, legumes, lean meat and eggs—we can use the remaining 20 per cent to indulge in whatever we want to enjoy that day. It's like a reward that we've earned for ourselves on the same day. Consequently, all binge eating, cheat meals and cheat days can be thrown out the window.

I first figured this out about a year ago, on my birthday. There were so many cakes at home that day, and I spent the morning indulging myself in them. By noon, I felt light-headed with the sugar overdose (remember I mentioned earlier how processed food makes you feel once you are done eating them?), so I decided to balance out the rest of my meals with simple and easily digestible food, giving lesser preference to the taste. I ate lots of veggies, had around five egg whites and a protein shake with a lot of water to hydrate myself well. Basically, what I was doing was crowding in my fibre and protein to crowd out the refined processed junk that I had eaten. The next morning, I felt much lighter, unlike when I usually eat a lot of junk and feel bloated for a few days.

Also, when I weighed and measured myself a few days later to casually check in, I had still managed to lose half a kilogram, and had even lost an inch from my waist, so I knew for sure that this wasn't because of muscle or water loss. It was much later that I understood the principle behind this, when I started reading more and came across the 80/20 rule that I follow! Now I use the 80/20 principle whenever I am on the maintenance phase, especially when I don't have any specific goals but just want to keep things going. I return to macro tracking when I have a specific goal of fat loss or muscle gain.

The one tip I want to give you before you start out is to focus more on the 80 and not too much on the 20—what you do 80 per cent of the times will determine the result that you are going to get. Eating healthy, regular exercise and getting enough sleep are what you need to prioritize in the week.

This 80/20 principle is simply based on estimation, for those of us who find it hard to track our macros consistently, so it's highly imperfect in that sense. In order to narrow down your margin of error, you need to be a little precise and have a system in place to do this. So how do you keep track of whether you are doing it right 80 per cent of the time? You write it down. You need to be able to look at it and evaluate it. Our mind has this amazing way of tricking us into believing that 80 per cent of the time we are doing the right things, but unless we have it written down we will never be able to keep track of where we are heading. I love using colours and highlighting the 80 (green) and 20 (red) in different colours in my journal, so when I see more red than green at the end of the day, I know that I need to work on the 80 per cent a lot harder on the next day. This is how I determine whether I am able to do the 80/20 principle justice. This is the only guidance here which helps me make better choices.

While we typically keep focusing on diet and exercise, those two alone will not help you drop your body fat. Including the environmental factors around you is also significant during this process, so we need to focus on:

1. Nutrition
2. Movement
3. Proactive stress reduction
4. Sleep rest and recovery

In each of these areas, you need to reflect on what you are doing, according to the 80/20 principle.

For example, let us look at stress reduction.

Lay out your goals to reduce stress. For instance, you might include:

- Journalling every day in the morning for 10 minutes.
- Recalling what caused you anxiety throughout the day every night before sleep, and working to dismantle the anxiety.

- Meditating and taking deep breaths every day for a couple of times.

When you reflect back on the week, and return to what you have written down, if you realize that you only meditated once and you missed out on journaling for a couple of times in the week, this record will help you understand that you only did 20 per cent of the work in this area. This will enable you to focus and perform better on stress reduction in the coming week for the benefit of your goals.

This applies the same way to your sleep, movement, physical activity and the rest you allow your body too. Eighty per cent of accuracy needs to be the aim. I used to maintain a journal consistently. It included the time when I would go to sleep, when I would wake up, a record of the days I trained and the days when I did not, my movement or step count on each day, my water intake, the days I meditated and the days where I skipped it, etc. For eating, I had a separate page where I once again used colour-coding to indicate the percentage of unhealthy food and healthy food that I consumed.

If you focus on 80 per cent efficiency in each of these categories, what do you think the overall effect will be? You will be living the dream lifestyle and supporting your body in the way it needs to get fit and healthy. That's how you apply the 80/20 rule in the most powerful way.

Occasionally, among my clients, I also find people who get extremely anxious about the 20 per cent relaxation that this plan advises, especially in the area of nutrition. To these people, who feel like the thought of eating whatever they want for 20 per cent of the time while on a calorie deficit plan stresses them out—like going out to eat ice cream—I feel that this method is not going to work. We might have to work on that stress and try to understand why such thoughts arise in the first place.

In spite of working and figuring out the root cause, there is still a certain group of people who like to stick to the idea of 'all or nothing'. They never want to have anything with sugar, because they consider it to be a bad food. It's not in their radar, they won't question it at all, and I actually see them doing better this way. This kind of determination might come from the understanding that if they are given an opportunity to indulge themselves in dessert, for example, they might begin with a small portion at first, but soon give in and uncontrollably consume larger and larger portions. Thus, to their minds, the 'all or nothing' approach actually has a positive impact, because it sets them up for a long-term plan and prevents them from deviating back and forth. It also takes away the guess work and the stress out of it for this category of people, since they do not even have to negotiate with themselves. But even to this group of people, the 80/20 principle cannot be applied only when it comes to food. With respect to the sleep, stress and movement, I still emphasize on what I've said before and ensure that the ones coached by me keep up with this ratio.

However, this is not what the average person is like. Most people I know, including myself, love the 80/20 rule because it allows us to figure out how to eat intuitively. If I am eating well at home for the most of the week, and if my friend invites me to watch a movie and then go out to eat, I don't hesitate anymore and simply go along with it. Once I finish enjoying the outing, I return home to my veggies. I love having that freedom. If and when it goes out of control, I ensure that I stop, look at the situation and evaluate what I have to do to get back on track.

So, for all of you who ask me if I'm just sharing photos of food that I don't eat on my Instagram stories . . . no, that's not what I do. That's not who I am! You can't have the cake and not eat it! Instead, you can have your cake . . . but just eat it without guilt and know how to handle it! That's my motto.

23

Do You Have the Guts to Fail?

I love to fail, and I look forward to failure. You heard that right.

I have realized with my share of experiences so far that failure, be it in life or in fitness, can be rewarding and inspiring in more ways than one. If taken in the right spirit, it can push your mind in a certain direction and enable optimum performance. I have personally benefited tremendously by understanding the psychology of failure and success while training to increase my performance capacity.

As someone who has been pretty hard on myself for everything that I do, I have felt the pain of failure several times in my life. The problem is that I used to feel like I had failed even when it was not necessary—for example, if everything did not work out the way I wanted, it would start affecting me. When I participated in a certain beauty pageant competition when I was 17 years old, I badly wanted to win the title at any cost, just like every other participant in it. For whatever reason, although I reached the finals, won three subtitles and was one among the top five out of twenty contestants, I didn't win the crown. I counted that to be a big failure. Given my age and lack of exposure at that time, instead of trying to understand what I lacked and how I could improve on that, I took the failure very personally, so much so that for many years after that, I disliked the very idea of competing against others and would refuse to entertain anyone who approached me about a contest or a competition. I think that failure mainly crushes your ego, and that's why we become people who dismiss everything blindly when something fails once or twice. I probably missed a lot of good experiences, and maybe I would have learnt quite a few skills and gotten better at handling the challenges of life early on, had I realized that it is not the end of the world when a certain door closes.

Remember how we all used to make a big deal as kids about our scores on tests? We were conditioned and pressured by our parents to feel that ranking first in class was of utmost importance. I think back on how I was an annoying student, especially how I behaved with my classmates, since I'd often try to find out if anyone who scored higher than me on a test had been accidentally given better marks than me. I feel ashamed and embarrassed that I was so obsessed with scoring the top grade. When I was in school, from class 8 onwards, I used to cry myself to sleep before each unit test, since I was afraid that I would fail even if I had prepared well for the test. Nobody told me the real truth, that it is not the academic grades, but the passion and willingness to work hard to achieve excellence that define one's success in life. These mundane failures that we see in day-to-day life don't matter in the larger scheme of things. If only I had known this back then!

Failure in a relationship with a friend, family member or relative is the most common kind of failure. Despite all our experiences and growth, most of us still can't come to terms with it. Even if you feel like you have not done anything wrong, it still feels like a terrible failure, one that especially hurts the ego, when you and that person can no longer continue and have to part ways. This is probably because we have several expectations of the people around us, and imagine that they'll all be our companions until death. When that doesn't work out, we tend to associate the failure of the relationship with a personal failing, and it is something that affects our future too. Even with friends, when we used to disagree about matters, I used to suppress my actual feelings and then blame myself for any arguments or differences. This has deeply affected my self-esteem. There were even times when I knew that I was at no fault for the failure of the relationship, but I'd still sit in my room and think about the ways in which I could set things right with that person, and if I'd ever be able to have a healthy relationship again and so on.

When my marriage failed, it shattered me completely. Like every girl, I too had the dream of getting married to someone, raising a family with that person and spending each moment of my life with my own family, sharing the happy and turbulent moments of life together. But life is certainly not going to go the way we want it to, and my marriage fell apart. I thought my entire life had failed when this happened. We all know how marriages are seen in our society, and my mind and heart were conditioned to feel that this was the end of everything. It crushed me. I didn't want to get out of my bed or do anything at all, and I used to just look at the ceiling for days on end, with my eyes tearing up all the time. I didn't want to talk to anyone nor sleep nor eat nor leave my room. I felt numb and dead.

But the one good thing about me is that I've never been someone who gives up easily. I'm a lot like my father in that way—he started from scratch, with no family background or wealth to back him up. My grandfather was a farmer in a remote village deep inside the district of Thanjavur, called Irandaam Pulikaadu, in Tamil Nadu. After his primary education in a government school, with Tamil as the only medium of instruction, he came to Chennai, learnt English, pursued Law and made it to the top with a lot of grit, resilience and perseverance, all on his own. My father was the advocate general of Tamil Nadu for a full term, when Dr Jayalalitha was the chief minister, and he is still a practising Senior Advocate at the Supreme Court and High Court at 75. He has successfully built a family and provided so much for my brother and me, with no help taken for all that he has achieved in life today. I admire him so much and feel motivated by his journey in all that I do in my own life.

I have also realized after much reflection that most things have not come easy to me, either in my career or in my life. Be it my popularity and celebrity status, or the kind of work that I get, things never fell into place like I've noticed it happening for other people. Have you noticed that there are some who, before we even realize it, skyrocket in popularity? This is something that people call 'overnight stardom'. The film industry gives this status to a few individuals, and I have no idea how it must be for that person to suddenly be placed on a pedestal with all that attention on them, after being in a bubble until that point. It must definitely be hard to handle in some ways, but it must surely be a great excitement too. Returning to myself, my career's trajectory has been similar to that of my father. I work hard, face rejections, stay motivated and keep on going until I finally achieve my dream, or things don't work out and something better comes along. I actually don't feel sad about this, because this process helps me grow stronger and learn a lot more than if I had achieved my goals quickly and easily.

When I began weight training, I started with a pair of 2.5 kg dumb-bells for 12 reps of squats. That was my strength level on day one. Today, I can lift close to 60 kg on a back squat with a barbell. When I'd started, I couldn't lift the bar at all, let alone attempt to bench press with the small bar (even without any weights on it). My knees would wobble and my form was terrible on a lunge or dead lift. When it comes to any kind of training, form is integral. If you don't have a good form through guidance and spotting, it can lead to irreparable injuries in the long run.

I failed, failed, failed. It was frustrating and disappointing for me to keep failing and seeing posts on social media by other colleagues in the gym who were performing better than me. But I didn't want to quit. I took this up as a challenge—I was going to learn, adapt and excel. I started focusing on my protein intake to build muscle in my body, which was probably not sufficient given the fact that I had inherited the vegetarianism of my ancestors. To my surprise, after a month I gradually started to see progress in the way I lifted and I could adapt to different weights as well. The same weight was also becoming slightly easier to lift, my form was getting better and my recovery was faster. I felt like I was winning this my way.

I failed, I learned, I failed again, and then I did better. I was finally able to see it working!

This was my first-ever breakthrough, and it gave me the motivation I needed to continue. As I started progressing with weights, I slowly developed the courage to lift even heavier weights, and to push my limits while being spotted to set the foundation right.

Alongside that, my mind started to feel happier too. When you're lifting heavy weights, your mind simply can't afford to wander. You need to focus 100 per cent on your breathing, form and technique, otherwise you're screwed. My muscles would feel so tired by the end of a workout that I had no choice but to rest, eat right and recover before the next session. As a result, the insomnia that had been plaguing me for weeks slowly started to resolve itself.

Wake up, eat, work out, nap, eat some more, work out again and sleep. This was my routine that entire time for about 6 months. My mind did not have the time or space to think about anything else. I was no longer even aware of what the world outside thought of me. I stopped thinking too much and hence, I stopped crying too much.

A significant portion of the credit for this mental change goes to the good friends who came as a blessing in my troubled times. They consistently made the effort to lift me up. This was when I realized the impact of real friends around me, and it helped me understand who would support me no matter what. If I didn't answer their texts, they would check in with one of my family members to ensure that I was fine. If I wanted to go out, all I needed to do was to tell them, and they would drop their work and show up for me. They never gave unsolicited advice or offered opinions on what they thought I should do, judged or discussed my problems behind my back. My friends were the most supportive people I could have asked for.

These days, I don't like to use the word 'failure' except when I'm talking about it in the context of fitness. When a certain relationship doesn't work out, it means that we have 'fallen out' over a difference in our thoughts, opinions or something else. It is not a failure.

The end of a relationship has often been described with words like 'separation', 'break-up' or 'divorce' by society. They are often made to seem like burdens which we need to carry for the rest of our lives. But in reality, the end of a relationship is as simple as the expiry date of a driving licence or passport. Since the world around us makes a big deal out of it, we feel burdened to add a huge amount of value to it. If we part ways with a person with whom we were deeply attached to in the past, do we miss the person or the memories we made with them? Isn't it the latter? When that person stops being a significant part of our lives, if we don't assign the same value and power to them as we had in the past, it won't feel like a great burden. At the end of the day, we all have one life. We are free to make our choices, and when a relationship does not work out the way we thought it would, we are free to part ways with people. I feel it is so much better to talk and get out of a relationship mutually when you don't feel involved in it anymore than to hang around in it for external factors, thereby making both your partner and you unhappy and making the whole family equation gradually dysfunctional. I would rather live alone and be happy than be in a committed relationship and feel lonely in it. This is just my opinion. Yours might be

different, and I am nobody to judge your opinion. To each
their own.

However, I do think that we all generally need to relax and
see the positive part of life and our failures. If we don't, they'll
just keep adding up as a burden on our shoulders, leaving
us with more and more baggage. The end of my marriage
has done a lot of good things to me as a person. I became
more sensitive, non-judgemental, more caring towards people
around me and felt more independent. I have been able to live
my life to the fullest and take decisions that I probably would
not have had the luxury to take if I wasn't single today. Failure
is indeed good, if you take it in the right sense.

Letter to Self

Dear Ramya,

Whatever has happened is in the past, and whatever is meant
to happen will happen too, whether you worry about it or
not. Now breathe and spend your energy on what you can
control. Live fully in this moment, because that's the only
thing that belongs to you.

Exercise:

Write a letter to yourself, with some words of motivation to
come back to when life knocks you down:

1. _____

2. _____

3. _____
4. _____
5. _____
6. _____
7. _____

24

Life Lessons I Learnt by Lifting Weights

What makes fitness so powerful?

I love going to the gym and training not only because of the way it helps me attain my body goals, but also for all the lessons that I learn which help me with my personal growth. It's not the kind of growth you get by reading a self-help book or going to a personality development class. I learn a lot about things that I am mostly unaware of. A lot of the people I coach tell me that the reason they join my Fitness Program or go to a gym is because they don't feel too good about the way they look. That's how I started out too! But it was only after I realized how working out changed my life that I felt the connection to show up and keep going. We face all sorts of challenges in our lives, from a family member passing away to huge crises at work, and I feel that my perspective about these has had its changes. Now, with my current mindset, I see such challenges adding value to my life, and this is what I owe to fitness. I'll explain this below in detail. Resilience to change becomes a part of you when you lift weights.

Now, here are the valuable lessons I have learnt by lifting weights.

1. My Relationship with Pain and Struggle Changed

This is something I learn every single day when I train.

Let's say I am doing a leg day training session, and I need to do 12 reps of a back squat loaded with weights on the barbell. When I had just started getting used to lifting weights, as I reached the 8th or 9th rep, the pain would kick in on my glutes, and this would be evident on my face too. I would often scream out and say that I couldn't finish doing it. I would feel sore afterwards, and since the soreness was something new as well, I would feel terrible and keep asking my trainer if something had gone wrong and complain about the pain to them. The way I handle this pain has evolved over the years.

Early on, working out was all about how I looked. After I started associating it more with muscle endurance and the health benefits that it provides, I realized that I can push myself through the pain. I figured that the pain was temporary—it was a necessary pain, to help grow my muscle, and since it was beneficial to my growth, I started to enjoy this kind of pain. Now, I am stretching my body's capacity to adapt, and I love that. If I had continued my job as an anchor, because I was told I was good at it, I liked it and was successful and made a lot of money from it, I would have never tried out other things in life and I would never know my body's capacity to survive newer challenges. I knew that moving on meant more work, putting myself in situations that I had never encountered before. That meant risk-taking, learning new things, failure and discomfort and so on. Had I not taken that chance and embraced my pain and attempt something out of my comfort zone, a career in the wellness or film industry would not have materialized for me. During the last two years, while coping with the pandemic, I was able to thrive in my career as a health coach by conducting online programs and workshops only because I had shifted things around earlier. Had I not done that, I would probably have been stuck at home waiting for opportunities in films and would have started to feel miserable about my situation. I would not have even written this book if I had not taken these decisive steps to change my life after I started training.

No matter who we are and how much money we have life is always going to make us encounter pain and challenges. You must and should seek help, confide in friends or family when you face physical or mental pain or a big challenge that you can't handle. In my case, getting comfortable with the physical soreness that results from training regularly led me to accept that pain is a part of life and we should look at it in that way.

This is why they say 'no pain no gain'!

2. Embracing Failure as Part of the Process

I want to paint a picture about failure by going back to my initial weight training days again, this time even before I had started lifting heavy weights. I was not able to squat regularly, let alone while using a dumb-bell, and I would always knock my knees. My posture was not good, I felt shaky and the whole idea of doing weights just did not feel right to me. I was pushing myself as much as I could to squat, but I was just not getting there. There are a few ways to tackle this when all of us attempt to train for the first time:

a.   We could say that we are done with it and give up.
b.   We could accept that this is just a part of the process and we are always going to experience this initial challenge. If we stop at this stage, our bodies won't change and all our efforts will go in vain.

Option 2 was the reason I scraped through those early days. I just kept focusing on the smaller steps and it got easier with each passing day.

Is failure a part of any process? It definitely is.

In fact, I used to have this inherent fear of attempting new things, whether it was to learn a new skill or to act on an idea, because I was afraid that I might fail. I would simply think about how cool it would be if I could do something that another person had already done, like starting a new business venture, opening a food stall, making my own short film and pitching it to other agencies and several other ideas like these which would never make it past the 'vision board' that I have at home. When I started training with weights and failing at a certain rep on a certain weight, but I was later able to do that exact weight on the exact rep that I'd failed with practice and practice, the entire process became easier and easier. All my practice and training taught me this: If I don't take a chance, how will I ever be able to find out what real answer awaits me? I envy people with businesses who try new things rather than just sitting and planning forever. They are capable of outperforming themselves, because of that instinct to try new things.

What happens if you don't sit and analyse your errors and instead try again and fail?

I don't care much about that now. What matters is that I at least tried—the attempt is worth knowing that I am not sitting around constantly thinking to myself, since I have done something to receive an answer, whether it works for me or not. If the attempt itself does not succeed I don't consider it to be a failure. For me, failure is only when I don't attempt something or don't learn from my experiences.

3. Learning to Care for Myself

This has taken me a real long time to realize. I have been someone who started working out not because I liked myself but because I didn't like myself. I overtrained, stressed myself out and was doing ridiculous dieting, and the irony of it all was that I had not made much progress with my physique because I wasn't treating myself properly. It took me a long long time to realize that I need to treat myself like how I would treat someone I love. I prioritized taking care of my body over caring about what other people thought of how I looked. This was around the time when I was punishing myself because I felt I was not putting enough work in and was constantly criticizing myself for it.

The day when I came home after an audition and looked into the mirror was when I had my realization. Once that had happened, my training and nutrition became appropriate,

I started treating my body well and adapting to what it communicated to me in terms of hunger, rest and recovery. The side effect of was that I started to feel like I looked better than before while looking at the same mirror.

I realized that when I was training and not caring for myself, but just chasing those results, I was overdoing it. I was always beating myself up for something and feeling fatigued all the time. Everything changed once I started treating myself well. If my gut didn't feel good, I would not be pushing on the protein requirement for muscle, but go easy on myself with more fluids and improve my digestive issues. When I felt exhausted, I would focus on sleep instead of training, and when I was too sore, I would go to the gym and work on mobility exercises to help me relax and stretch out the muscles rather than rushing to burn more calories.

4. Learning to Chase the Things I Can Change and Letting Go of Those I Cannot

I have hardly heard anyone saying they love their body the way it is. How many of us constantly keep complaining day in and day out about the way our body parts are shaped? People think they are too fat or short or thin and so on—we are so focused on what we don't have that it is hard to realize that we might never get exactly what we seek because our genetics might not allow it. In my case, it is getting flat abs with the definition visible. When I almost attained that a couple of years back, the other parts of my body started looking so weak and fragile that I knew I would not be able to sustain the look for long and it compromised my overall physique. Genetics and our body structure also play a role in what we can achieve. Some goals will be either unrealistic or unachievable, so we must focus on what we can achieve with our body.

I struggle with different goals at different points in time. While glancing at an Instagram post by an athlete or an international fitness trainer, I would often desire to have a similar frame. For example, don't we all love the South Indian diva Simran even today for her rock-solid abs and that waistline? Every woman I know envies her secretly for her curves that she flaunts especially while she dances. I am no exception. I used to long for that too and Google what Simran eats, how she works out, etc., and tried to replicate that. And now I know that while I can put in the work needed to achieve my goals, it's not realistic to expect to have the exact same result as another person when it comes to my body. This lesson has taught me that it is important to accept who I am—my body type and my genetics, my bone structure and framework—and also focus on the strength that I can summon within my abilities. For example, I struggle to gain muscle, and no matter how hard I try, the muscles don't visibly show the way I'd like them to. This is not just due to my ancestry, but also the pitfalls of the vegetarian diet that I follow which can't match with all the essential amino acids one can get in a diet with animal protein (my dear vegans I feel you and as upsetting as it is, we have to address the deficiencies of our plant-based diet).[1] On the contrary, endurance-building workouts come

---

[1] https://impacttheory.com/episode/dr-gabrielle-lyon-2/; https://chriskresser.com/how-protein-supports-your-muscle-health-with-dr-gabrielle-lyon/#The_Problem_with_the_Vegan_Narrative; https://twitter.com/drgabriellelyon/status/1485635328857702405.

easier to me, and I feel that that is my strength too. My stamina helps me do movement and agility-based activities a lot easier than others, also because of my frame and because I practise different forms of training.

The lesson here is not only to accept it when things don't work the way we want them to, but also to be grateful for our strengths and use them to our advantage.

5. Perfect Doesn't Exist

Fitness can go in two different directions, and I have seen both ends of this. While it can go in a positive direction, which is what I am discussing here, the other side of it can be pretty traumatic with extreme dieting, surgeries, anabolic steroids, fat burners and things that are extremely unhealthy and potentially fatal. This pursuit can become very destructive if you don't have the right approach. I have mentioned my experiences along this journey in the earlier chapters of this book.

The negative path is commonly taken by people in showbiz who consider their body to be everything that they have and tend to feel deeply insecure even if they look incredible in the eyes of people who watch them. The fitness professionals we see in competitions, who try to perfect the way they look, fall into this bottomless pit, and so do the obese individuals who feel that their weight is the reason why they aren't happy and that losing it is the answer to all their current problems.

Truthfully, any goal or achievement in fitness or health will make us happy only when we have reached self-acceptance.

I have been in all the situations that I have mentioned above, and each time I would achieve a certain goal, I would not feel happy at all. I would want to do the next best thing for my body. It was when the formula was flipped, i.e. understanding that a happy state of mind would help me get fit, that things started working. Chasing perfection is simply a trap.

6. Being Humble

Fitness and being humble? It doesn't sound like these two can be interlinked, right? But they definitely are.

In fitness, there is always going to be someone who is stronger, fitter and even more knowledgeable than you and me. Whether I worked out in the smallest gym in my area at a time when most gyms were shut, or whether I competed in prestigious powerlifting competitions at a state level, there were always people that I saw around me who looked great and trained even more intensely than I did. In the case of some, their warm-up routines would be as intense as lifting my heaviest weight. All of that helped make me humble.

My dear fans and friends keep feeding my ego whenever I need it, and I am so grateful for that. But I am always humbled by the world of fitness, and I think it is a good thing because it keeps me learning and growing. I even have days when I would want to lift very heavy weights and end up getting buried under them at the gym! It is frustrating when I know that I can squat 50 kg easily, since I've done that in the past, but probably because of the gap in training or my lack of sleep or poor energy levels, I will not be able to do as much as I want—that realization is very humbling. Another observation that I've made is that as you get older, you need to put in additional work that is required to keep up with the same momentum of how you used to perform while exercising. It would be silly if I tried to compete with a 15-year-old in sprinting without warming up my body enough. This would not have been the case if we were of the same age. This too is a humbling lesson.

All of this is applicable in life too.

As an anchor, I have hosted hundreds of live shows/events/tv shows, and I have had my share of experiences when I would try to excel at my job by hosting events right after returning from another city or by participating in back-to-back shoots of different programmes on the same day. This would regularly backfire, and I would often feel dissatisfied and low on energy with my performance. Instead of looking for excuses and blaming everything around me, I started to analyse why this would occur. If I asked myself, how did I get here? I would know deep down that I was at fault. I should not have accepted to do multiple events on that day, or I should have requested to get the scripts in advance so that I could plan things out instead of racing to keep up with things in the last moment.

I think as long as I stay with fitness and weight training, this lesson will be a constant reminder for me. It's never going to leave me, and that is just how I want it to be.

7. Consistency over Strategy

We all wish for financial success and wish to lead a comfortable life. How can we achieve this?

The answer is: work hard, save your money and plan it on investments, don't go into debt and build on multiple sources of revenue.

This is simple enough in writing, at least. If I keep doing these every single day, I can be sure that I am on the right path to get what I want financially.

This applies in the fitness world too. A consistent person doing an average workout will get a better shape over time than somebody who follows the best workout regimen with the best trainer in the world but is inconsistent.

This takes me back to the time when my workouts were all aimed at one thing—burning loads of calories during the session. Now I have transitioned to showing up in the first place, checking in with myself to see how I feel on that day, and even if I don't feel it in me to push myself during the session, I still count the movements I do while training as something that I am progressing towards.

In my own relationships, I have seen that it is the little things, like wishing someone a good morning or sending a message to check in with people once in a while, that makes me feel more connected to the person over grand gestures of sending flowers or cakes once a year on my birthday.

8. The Journey Is More Important Than the Destination

When I got a job as a television host on a big channel a decade ago, the biggest source of happiness and excitement for me was that my job would help me meet and interview the actors I had watched while growing up. Being so rooted in Tamil cinema and having watched film after film upon release, this was only natural. Thus, I wanted to meet those actors, be able to host film promotions, attend preview shows for their films and take pictures with every single one of them so I could put the photographs up on my wall for me to admire.

I joyfully went about doing this. It worked out exactly how I had wanted it to. I would regularly take pictures of them and pin them up on the board that I hung in my room. It got crowded with photographs in no time, with innumerable photos ranging from A-listers to new entrants at several shoots, audio launches, award shows, star nights and so on.

While this was a very happy experience, my point is that I was always concerned about what to do next. I realized that my actual desire was to meet the people that I had idolized, and not to take endless pictures of them. It was more memorable to live in the moment with them and find out about their personal sides and have a connect with them—that was more fulfilling than the photographs that I took for my momentary satisfaction.

It is the same principle when we prepare for an exam too. We burn the midnight oil, study very hard, memorize as much as we can, give the exam and then immediately move on to something else. Even years after all of that, do we not tend to remember more about the experience of preparing for the exam than the questions and the answers.

9. Healthy Self-Criticism

I feel that self-criticism is not always negative. While we don't have to think things like 'I'm terrible and ugly', I personally also don't like to feel that 'I am perfect and nothing needs to change'. I like to be somewhere in the middle when it comes to this, so that I can look in the mirror and say that I objectively haven't been treating my body well, that I need to work on my posture a little bit and maybe I need to focus on those as my next goals. Being self-aware gives me the room for improvement. And no, this is not coming from a place of insecurity. It is simply like an inventory—I look back to my last few days or weeks to understand how I have been spending my time. Every time after a cutting phase, I go all out and splurge on food without training for a bunch of weeks. This observation, from a non-judgemental perspective, would then make me feel motivated to come back and improve on a certain goal, build some mobility after focusing only on lifting, eat better quality food and getting to my maintenance calories and so on. In life, this comes in handy when I know that I have made a mistake, and instead of brushing it under the carpet and pretending like it never happened, with this lesson in place I reflect on my problems, own up to my mistakes and find a solution without being hard on myself. If I have an argument with a colleague, friend or family member, which has become rare in recent times, I first analyse the situation from a neutral standpoint to discover why it happened. I try to consider other perspectives and examine myself from the outside to figure out why I crossed certain thresholds, and then work on how to handle similar situations in the future.

10. Finding the Balance

If there is no balancing while lifting weights—be it a dumb-bell, barbell or kettlebell—your core won't get stronger and you won't develop your body. Furthermore, you run the risk of getting injured. Balancing with weights is the basis of training. Time and again, what we have realized is that hard work and consistency can get us to our goals, but we need a certain balance to keep things stable and maintain our discipline.

How is this a life lesson? Well, we all need balance in our lives. Only focusing on one thing rarely works—when I focused on just building my physique, I was terribly unhappy and felt like I had a void inside of me all the time. I did not know what was missing until I started making an effort to strike out a balance in every area of my life—health, career, relationships and spirituality. I also keep one whole day of the week free, no matter how busy my schedule gets, to put the phones away and focus on my own needs. This was something I started doing only after joining The Institute of Integrative Nutrition (IIN, New York) for my Health Coaching Program that I undertook there. It was quite an awakening for me, as a big part of their holistic curriculum dealt with listening to my inner voice and keeping it alive.

I feel like our life is a constant dance that we perform, and in order to keep one area of our lives fulfilled, we tend to lose our balance and ignore another aspect. To achieve great things does take a lot of sacrifice, discipline and consistency, but in order to maintain it for a long time, we need that balance. It has taken me a very long time to figure this out and know how to weave around all of this.

25

Travel Hacks

'I have an early morning flight'.

'I have a late night flight'.

'I'm constantly working while travelling and can't take time off to stay fit'.

'I feel so jet-lagged living out of suitcases all the time'.

Those of you who travel frequently might be thinking along these lines. This is one of the biggest issues to address: when you have the drive to stay fit but are unable to because of practical difficulties.

If you have a job that makes you travel frequently, it is a challenging situation for sure. Being consistently health conscious when you are staying in a hotel, living on outside food, dealing with time zone differences and the lack of workout equipment (not all hotels have gyms, and if they do, some are limited to just a few treadmills) are few of the several factors that have made it difficult for me when I travel for shoots. Overcoming these problems requires planning strategically and figuring out a way to sustain your training.

The importance of movement at such times is significant. Moving around consciously, walking, taking the stairs, getting down from the car beforehand and looking for ways to rise up from a sitting position, fidgeting while sitting and even small movements (shaking, bending, rolling the neck from one side to another, stretching out) help over time. I have noticed a huge change on days when I move more (it helps me focus more, gives me more energy, I read my lines with more clarity and feel more confident while performing) compared to the days when I stay inside, shutting myself in the vanity van until it's time to walk in for a shoot.

Earlier, I did try researching the hotels I am supposed to stay at, booking a day pass at a gym near the hotel if the hotel gym isn't good enough and so on, but that never worked because it was too much effort. After tiring myself out from booking hotels and passes, I would end up without the motivation to go at all, and I would just want to flop onto the bed in the hotel, order food from room service and watch TV.

Just staying active is the most successful method during vacations. There is a benefit to moving around, of course, but when I want to hit certain difficult goals during the time of my shoots, I have to take it up by a notch and design a plan that has more structure to help me cater to my goals. When there is a time crunch and I only have about 30 minutes in my hotel room before heading out for the day, I am compelled to make use of it as effectively as possible and opt for a quick HIIT routine in the area next to the bed. The other solution is to ramp up the volume and intensity of training when I am in town, alongside less training without the equipment, but still structured effectively, while travelling. I always encourage my clients to continue the coaching programme with me and not take a full break when they travel, and they usually return baffled at how this proved to be the most impactful for them. It's one thing to reduce the intensity of your movement, but when you stop everything completely because of travel, you lose that momentum and it's hard to start again from where you left off.

Let's address this step by step, on how to stay on track with your health goals when you are on the road.

Workout

When I was shooting for my Telugu film recently in Coonoor and then in Hyderabad for about 20 days at a stretch, I had a proper training programme sent to me by my trainer, which included three full-body workouts. I looked up the hotel that had been booked for me, and on reaching I sent a video to my trainer of the equipment at the hotel's gym. My goal was to maintain the lean frame that I had, as my character in the film was a young girl in her mid-twenties, about to get married and I wanted my look to match that. My training in Hyderabad was high volume and highly intense (with access to a good hotel gym there), according to what my trainer sent me each day. It included three focused sessions per week that targeted all the muscles, and if I had extra time, my fourth day was a combination of core obliques along with high-interval training cardio, where I alternated between jogging for a minute, sprinting for a minute and walking for a minute on the treadmill for 45 minutes. However, when I was in Coonoor, I used to go for a nice and long 60-minute morning uphill walk and the lovely cold weather and picturesque natural views made it very blissful for me start the day on a great note.

I agree that it's harder to feel the motivation to work out when you are elsewhere on work and in a new city. On several occasions, I used to feel like skipping the gym afterwards because I wanted to go shop around or have dinner with friends. I started planning my workouts around the 45 minutes that I had in the morning. I wasn't eating breakfast at the hotel anyway, so instead of simply laying around in the bed, all I had to do was to wake up and jump out of the bed and go to the gym before my mind started wandering. Once I reached the gym, simply seeing all the other hotel guests exercising there was enough for me to get started. You could try this out too. Just act on it without giving yourself the time to think. There were also days when I took a break from the gym routine, when I just wore my trackpants and did a nice stretch routine and meditation in the morning before the shoots. On some days when I decided to go to the bazaar, I ensured I got a decent number of steps in with long walks.

If the shoot happened to be in a remote village, like the time I had to film for *Sangathalaivan*, I would simply do a full-body weight routine in my room. I realized that one can get really creative with the body weight workouts by doing the following.

a. Manipulating the tension in the muscle—for example, if you do 10 fast squats and then hold the squat position for 30 seconds without getting up. No matter how strong you are, these isometric static exercises can be quite intense, and the benefits one gets are pretty close to using weights. The other good thing here is that as I'm someone who resorts to traditional dumb-bell and barbell weight training back at home, when I do a full-body no-equipment workout while travelling, it sort of excites me and my body since it is newer and unfamiliar.

b. Using tempo speeds to squeeze and burn the muscle—for example, a push-up where you do it with slow negatives of 2–3 seconds and pause for each rep makes you put more emphasis on the back and the chest, and it activates those muscle fibres more strongly than the old-school resistance training workout.

I find these workouts so valuable because they are very short, I don't have to go anywhere to do them, they're novel, and very easy to commit to. There is no excuse for me to come up with when I can do these if I wake up and hit the gym immediately. Even if I miss them in the morning, I could still do them during the lunch break or in the evening after the shoot.

On the days when doing the conventional routine of exercising just didn't feel right, I'd listen to my body. For example, when I'd film for a song all day long, I would be dancing and working out during the shoot anyway. On those days, I would not overdo it, and probably do some stretches or walk or jog outside in the morning before the shoot.

I pack a pair of sneakers and tees, tracks and shorts wherever I go. They not only come in handy, but more importantly, they are also extremely comfortable to wear while travelling. This way, no matter what situation I am in, I can just keep walking to feel active.

Sitting in one place in a fixed position for a long time used to make me feel stiff and aggravate my body aches severely when I used to travel. Neck pain, back pain and shoulder pain were very regular during the long flights. Then I started doing these priming movements—I was ideally supposed to do them at least once a week while I was back at home to improve my posture, but I had completely neglected them then. Thus, during my trips, just before boarding the plane and while I was in the car, or just before I sat down to do my make-up, I did these movements. They have been very beneficial, and have improved the condition of my body. These priming movements have also helped my body respond better to static positioning for long durations.

Nutrition

Travelling also challenges my eating habits. It is harder than usual to eat right when I'm on the go, especially to make the right choices to eat when my sleep is unsteady and my workload it too much. But when I exercise, more often than not, I have observed that I tend to choose meals smartly. This is because when I work out every day, I am in the mindset to take care of my body, so I feel better and that also makes me more self-aware. I pay attention to hydrating myself frequently during the shoots and make other healthy choices.

While nutrition can't get anywhere close to perfection while travelling, I carry food items that can be handy to me even on the difficult days to help me stay on track. Some of these would be almonds that I can soak in water to eat in the morning, nut butters made at home that would be an ideal snack, my travel AeroPress and coffee powder to make coffee on my own whenever and wherever I want (you have to do this to understand what a blessing it can be), a few scoops of protein powder, protein bars and *makhanas* (lotus seeds) to snack on. If I have a long schedule, I get some oats, chia seeds, milk and fruits locally, and make my oats overnight with my recipe, and eat them as one of the meals (breakfast or dinner). The other standard meal for me when I travel would be soup and omelette with veggies if I stay in a hotel, and 99 per cent of the times that is what happens. With two meals sorted out, all I have to work on is lunch. Lunch is mostly provided by the production crew if I am filming, and I would have dal and a combination of 3-4 types of greens and veggies during lunch when I work. Rice is too heavy and makes me feel groggy. I try and eat smaller portions, but more frequently, if eating while travelling, a fruit or protein bar is my go-to snack.

When on a vacation, going a little off-track is totally understandable. But if you are completely unmindful, think about all the hard work that goes down the drain and how you'll need to put in twice the amount of effort when you return. I also indulge myself while travelling. I am a foodie and willingly give in when someone tells me that I must try a certain dish. I don't feel bad after eating these days, only because I don't do it too frequently for it to sidetrack me from my programme. Staying mindful is the single most important thing that keeps my nutrition steady while travelling.

Stay Hydrated

Puffy eyes, dry skin and lips—have you ever had these symptoms when out of a flight? The air inside of an aeroplane is extremely dehydrating because it is maintained in a certain way by the air-conditioning, thus sucking the moisture from your skin. The air pressure, on the other hand, resulting from the altitude, causes the body to hold water. The combination of these means that you retain water inside but lose lots of water from the skin.

The effects are temporary, fortunately. Once you get to sea level and have a meal, you'll be fine. Water retention generally clears overnight too. But I've gotten into the habit of drinking lots of water and applying generous amounts of moisturizer with sunscreen before getting on a flight. It has greatly helped in ensuring that I feel energetic right after getting off the flight (when you normally find people yawning and exhausted), and has also helped me look better. I usually take the early morning flight and rush to a shoot location straight from the airport to start working, so I don't feel the need to yawn and can't afford to look tired during the shoot.

Also, I normally carry an empty bottle in my handbag and refill it with water wherever I go, instead of spending money on water. If you're the type of person who forgets to drink water regularly, here are some tips that have helped me:

- Set an alarm to drink water every hour, or download an application on your mobile that will remind you to drink water.
- Drink water when you wake up, before or during your workout, and every time you go to the bathroom.
- Spice it up with lime, mint leaves and cut fruits.
- Get into the habit of drinking herbal tea or green tea at least twice a day.
- Eat water-rich foods such as watermelon, cucumber, tomatoes, etc.

Sleep

I cannot compromise on my beauty sleep during a trip. Between all my activities and constant moving about, my body is exhausted as it is, so ruining my sleep means amplifying this to another level. While it's harder to get a good night's rest when you're in a new space, a good tip that I can give you after working on it myself is to tire yourself out physically by being active throughout the day. This works like magic. If I don't sleep enough, it reflects on my work, focus, productivity, moods and so on, so after seeing its consequences, I absolutely do not compromise on sleep, especially when I have to travel for work.

Even when I am on a holiday and am just going with the flow, while I may not manage eight hours of sleep at a stretch, I try taking several naps during the flight (I do this all the time and not only does time fly by, but you also reach your destination fresh and well-rested) or while sitting in the car (needless to say, do this only when you aren't driving!). If you have to, excuse yourself from any boring meetings, find a cozy spot and doze off for a while (but don't forget to set an alarm on your phone for 10–15 minutes later, as you don't want to get caught by your boss!).

Keep Calm and Relax

There's no point rushing and trying to keep up with a packed itinerary if I don't feel rested or enjoy the moment while I live in it. Whatever my purpose or trip is, I pace myself by taking 10 minutes out in the morning or at night for silence and solitude. I just think and reflect on my day, the new people I met, my work on that day, the new place that I am visiting and what I learnt that day.

Beating the heat and the tiring sun by swimming in the hotel's pool is another good way to relax when on a vacation. If I am with a group of friends, we try playing an outdoor sport in the evenings—like badminton or volleyball.

These are optional tips, but they can also help while travelling.

1. Pack healthy snacks: I'm not suggesting that you meal prep and carry *dabbas* filled with food for the next two days. I am simply suggesting that carrying a small box of snacks, nuts, protein bars, fruits and nut butters instead of eating chips, samosas, biscuits and chocolates—things that one would be tempted to buy (at an exorbitant price) and munch on when hungry and travelling—is a good idea.

2. Head to the local grocery or fruit shop: I don't know about you, but this is my favourite part of travelling, no matter where I go. I head to a reasonably good supermarket on the first day of my trip just to pick up something healthy, find out what's available there (something that isn't available back in Chennai), and get some local fruits and curd. Sometimes, if there's a toaster in the room I'm staying in, or if I'm at an Airbnb or serviced apartment, I buy a few things and try my hand at cooking. It is so fulfilling to make my own meal when I'm outside home. It is also very healthy!

3. Walk it out: Every year, when I go to Kodaikanal, I rent a bicycle and jog around the lake too. Also, while

sightseeing and doing local tours, if Google Maps tells me that it will take less than 25 minutes to walk back to my hotel, I choose that over taking a cab back after dinner. Ditch the local transport—I have realized that you can explore much more in a new place when you develop the habit to start walking. Walking is not just about weight. It helps to reduce stress, helps with your heart's health, helps your lungs to fill up with good oxygen if it is an outdoor walk and it gets you the vitamin D you need among other things—so I just don't think twice when it comes to walking.

Whether you're travelling for work or fun, you should never lose your focus on yourself. So prioritize yourself by staying fit!

26

Skin Food and Haircare

Skincare

Almost everybody who meets me compliments me on my complexion. The truth is, I haven't done much to take credit for this. For the most part, it is the direct blessing of good genes from my parents. But to ensure that I don't reverse that, my contribution to keep it going has been following a certain regimen in a disciplined way. I don't do much experimentation on my skin and leave it the way it is. I focus on healing the skin and hair from within the body rather than using superficial creams that aren't long-lasting. Everyone's skin is different, and instead of blindly following home remedies, understanding my body through the years and knowing what suits and doesn't suit me has been incredibly useful in this regard. My skincare routine is formed on the recommendations of my dermatologist Dr Renita Rajan, based on my work, exposure to pollution, my skin type and other associated factors. I don't experiment with my skin.

Understanding My Reaction to Dairy

A lot of talk these days is about dairy and its connection to the skin and gut health. After noticing the changes it had on my friends who had recently turned vegan, I decided to give this a shot, just to see the difference. While you may know that I have decent skin, I also need to tell you that I have sensitive and problematic skin too. I deal with constant redness and inflammation under exposure to heat and lights. Even wearing new jewellery or using a skin cream or a new deodorant agitates my skin. My skin is prone to acne as well. Just avoiding dairy made my skin clear up, and that feeling of uneasiness in my stomach vanished.

Milk is meant to be given to infants in the form of breast milk from the mother, to supply the initial dose of nutrients that they need. It is believed that drinking raw cow's milk from, which is meant for calves, can create health issues in humans due to the harmful pathogens present in it.[1] While our elders tell us to drink milk with the best of intentions—for the purpose of strengthening our bones and improving our calcium intake—the milk that we drink today has several fillers and antibodies. That is the enemy here, more so than the milk itself, which makes most of us develop lactose intolerance.

Being a vegetarian, it is difficult to give up on the entire dairy family, and while I am lactose intolerant (since it is an ingredient in milk), I am not dairy intolerant yet. However, I do limit dairy as much as possible.

---

[1] https://www.ncbi.nlm.nih.gov/pmc/articles/PMC3882853/.

Also note that if dairy is harmful for us, it'll mean that we need to reduce consuming, if not stop altogether, all dairy products—that includes chocolate, ice cream, pizza, pasta and everything which requires milk in recipes. Though I am a huge fan of chocolate, just limiting the amount of baked sweets I have and resorting to 75 per cent dark chocolate have worked well for me.

If you want to try this out for yourself, I suggest that you try going on a dairy elimination diet after consulting with your physician first. I have to warn you that the first five days will be a bit hard, and you might have some withdrawal symptoms like headache, nausea, cravings for dairy and light-headedness, but remember that this is all an indication that things are progressing in the right direction. To compensate for the loss of dairy, crowd in more fruits and vegetables in your meals. You can find substitutes for cow's milk or even make almond, oat or soy milk easily at home. Watch my YouTube video on the 'Stay Fit With Ramya' channel to know the steps to make vegan milk at home. By the end of three weeks, you will see and feel a difference. After that, you can reintroduce one food at a time for a few days to check if it is only a specific food that is your problem or if it is the entire dairy family. For example, start with paneer and have it for 3–4 days and observe. If you feel fine, proceed to curd for another 3–4 days, then cheese and finally milk. The food that is messing with your system can be spotted and removed in this way, while you get to have the other by-products that were not causing any issues. Having said this, I am not saying everyone has to go off dairy too. These days the number of people with dairy intolerances is high so it's good to test it out once. If you feel you are ok, you can continue with your dairy normally.

Handling Acne

Acne is a regular problem I have to deal with, as my T-zone is naturally more sensitive and oilier than the rest of my face. As a result, pimples pop up every now and then, owing to stress, heat, excessive sweating, hormonal changes and the make-up products I use.

Over time, I have realized that stressing out is the worst thing to do in such situations. Stress makes the acne stubborn and resistant. No amount of sandalwood paste or acne creams help then! Instead, I take deep breaths, relax and consciously increase my water intake.

Washing my face 3–4 times a day with cold water also helps when I get acne. I simply use aloe vera gel to moisturize my face after that. I have tried some creams that advertise that they will solve the acne problem, but usually they just worsen it for me.

I also avoid waxing and threading of eyebrows and the upper lip during this time. I simply avoid increasing further risks to my already super sensitive skin during the acne season. For hair removal, only laser hair removal has worked for me. Waxing was giving me itching, redness and heavy inflammation, and I used to dread the feeling but still put up with it until my doctor changed it to laser hair removal.

The real tip I can give you here is to go to a good dermatologist in your city, because after examining your skin, they can devise a treatment that is ideal for you. I understand that a lot of us feel reluctant to check with doctors for every small problem, but that is the only way to get a permanent solution, and they will show good results in a short time if you follow the doctor's instructions properly.

Lemon Water/ACV/ABC Juice on an Empty Stomach

This is a tricky one. In the past, I have had lemon water after waking up, and have even been someone who used to rub lemon peels on my hands. I have luckily gotten away with it, but this is not the same for everyone. Lemon juice is highly acidic, and its effects vary from person to person. Using lemon for your skin has its own advantages and disadvantages. Lemon can be an irritant to the skin for some and help remove tan for some others. Do your research on the ingredients that will be safe for your skin and then go about using them. Remember that 'natural' doesn't automatically mean that it's safe to use all the time. As for ABC juice, it's just one of the fashionable ways of introducing the different colours into your diet sustainably, and when you start drinking it as part of your regimen, it gives you good skin, hair, nails and an overall vitamin and mineral boost.

Dark Circles

My biggest problem with my skin are the dark circles that I tend to develop under my eyes when I'm sleep-deprived after continuous shoots, stress or anxiety. I'm done with trusting the under-eye creams or gels for dark circles, for I have tried everything and have found nothing that works for me. For my dark circles, the only thing I can resort to is sleep, and I swear by it. This sleep can neither be once or twice a week, nor at different timings on different days. When I have a sleep routine, if I wake up and go to sleep at regular times even when I don't sleep peacefully, my sleep is adequate enough for me to see a change in my dark circles.

Another perennial issue that I was born with is eye puffiness. Whether I sleep too much or too little, my eyes look tired and puffy when I wake up on most days. People say that eye puffiness can be due to water retention, so these days, I try to limit my salt intake as much as I can. Increasing the amount of water I drink helps. In addition to this, I also keep tea bags (that have been refrigerated) under my eyes. Potato slices, cucumber slices and ice cubes also work decently well.

Removing My Make-Up before Going to Bed

No matter how late it is when I return home after a shoot, or how tired I might be, I always make it a point to remove my make-up completely before hitting the sack. To remove the dirt and make-up from the face and eyes completely, I use virgin coconut oil. If there is an ongoing acne issue, however, I use cleaning lotion (Cetaphil is ideal for any skin). After completely wiping myself clean, I wash again with a gentle face wash—right now, I use Avène's cleansing foam, which works for my skin.

Avoiding Salon Treatments

I don't enjoy parlour facials and bleaches as much, or applying anything that is chemical-based on my skin. I believe that these can have irreversibly harmful effects on the skin. Since my skin is very sensitive and doesn't respond well to most treatments, I often end up having burns, redness, itchiness and breakouts. If I want my skin to look fresher, I consult my dermatologist and she works on a safe, customized skincare ritual for me. I cannot stand facial massages, pinching, rubbing or touching the face either!

Keeping a Tab on My Vitamin D Levels

One more thing I want to caution you about is the vitamin D deficiency that most of us suffer from. Since we all tend to hide ourselves from the sun and spend most of our time indoors, this is an extremely common problem. We need to expose ourselves to the sun by regularly going on brisk morning walks at the right time, doing sun salutations and letting the sun seep into our body periodically. Alternatively, you could take vitamin D supplements and shots depending on your physician's advice. Exposure to the sun is vital to your overall health and well-being. Soaking up those rays can ward off depression, strengthen your bones, and even help regulate your blood pressure. Timing matters and ensure you do it early morning or late evening.

Sunscreen

Too much of sun exposure and harsh radiations to ultraviolet rays can damage your skin and that is why sunscreen should be used every single day. I remember that was the only thing Dr Renita told me to do when I asked her eagerly for an a.m.

and p.m. routine for young and supple complexion. She also warned me that I would be increasing the risk of skin cancer and early skin aging by not using sunscreen. So no matter the season, or the weather, skip all your other skincare products if you want, but never the sunscreen. When it comes to picking the right sunscreen, again you need guidance on what would work effectively for your skin type. Just like I get help from my skincare expert, do seek guidance before you select your sunscreen.

Skin Foods

I recommend using vitamin C, hydration and good fats for the glowing dewy skin that we all want.

The checklist I follow for this is:

- Drink about 3–4 litres of water every day.
- Eat at least two servings of fruits a day—oranges, strawberries, guavas, apples, etc. one of which will be rich in vitamin C
- Eat almonds in the morning and two walnuts in the evening (omega fatty acids work very well for the skin).
- Avoid sugar and milk as much as possible.
- Stay away from processed food and fried snacks.

Haircare

I am often asked how I take care of my hair while exercising. We tend to lose hair while we exercise because scalp sweating can dry out the scalp, thereby impeding hair growth. The natural salts present in sweat affect the colour of your hair too, and can cause premature greying. Let's not forget how sweaty hair can ruin a great hairdo and alter the natural scent of the hair follicles.

While washing hair everyday isn't necessarily a good or bad thing, I wash my hair once every two days, and when it's feeling particularly sweaty I simply wash it off even if that means I have to wash it every day.

I normally tie my hair in a firm high bun or pull it back into a low ponytail while working out. It prevents the sweat from seeping into the deeper areas of my hair. I also find that my hair is easier to comb and untangle from a bun. I do like the idea of braids for a workout too, because when you unbraid it later, you get a nice texture too. All of this is strictly something that I do just before working out, for if I tie up my hair tightly at all times the roots lose their strength and the scalp starts thinning due to that. I also wear a cap when I step out for a walk under the sun.

At night, I use a scrunchie to tie my hair in a loose bun, or braid my hair loosely to prevent any kind of breakage while sleeping.

My shampoo and conditioners are sulphate free and recommended by my doctor. With the constant styling and heating products that my hair gets exposed to due to filming, I keep it minimalistic on all the other days even if that means allowing my wet hair to dry naturally and not using a hairdryer. That is the break or the rest period for my hairline to recover from the overdose of chemicals.

It is not wise to use our skin or hair as a guinea pig by constantly experimenting with gimmicks that we read about on the Internet. I used to often colour my hair, keep changing hair texture with smoothening and straightening treatments earlier, but after seeing the hair fall and breakage that comes along with it, now I don't get tempted to try these out anymore unless my work requires it. And the one rule that I now follow and recommend is that when you are in doubt, ask the experts.

You are all you really have, and I feel that you have to love yourself the most.

It's amazing how much the surface of your skin can reveal about what's going on in your gut. That way, our skin and hair are great at telling us when something may be off balance internally. There is a lot of research currently going on regarding gut health and how the make-up of gut bacteria is linked to every health issue we have. Remember that while we aren't born with bad skin or hair—most times it has a lot to do with our unhealthy lifestyles and unhygienic practices. You don't have to punish yourself by restricting yourself from eating your favourite foods entirely, but good skin and hair starts with a good gut. The next time you see a pimple, dark circles under your eyes, inflammation, puffiness or hair fall remember there is a high chance of it being connected to your food intake, your stress levels, your sleep cycle and more. Also, no amount of beauty tips and home remedies can help unless you solve the root cause of that problem; when you have an issue, stop experimenting with random things and please visit an experienced professional and ask for guidance.[2]

---

[2] https://www.dermatologytimes.com/view/gut-bacteria-linked-to-inflammatory-skin-disease.

Frequently Asked Questions

1. I am content with the way I look, except for my
   tummy/thighs/butt/hands/bust. How do I lose weight
   just there?
   You cannot control where you lose fat. Spot reduction
   cannot happen, so don't fall prey to such claims and false
   marketing. When you lose a percentage of your total
   body fat, your body will also naturally lose fat in the
   places where you particularly intend to lose it—maybe
   first there, if you are lucky, or maybe last, that's for
   the body to decide, not you or me! This is a gradual
   process and needs a lot of patience and consistency.
   Also, stubborn fat is something that has been deposited
   over years of following a bad lifestyle with unhealthy
   eating habits, and it will take time to go. So, be mentally
   prepared to stay calm, consistent and most importantly,
   be kind to yourself.

2. Will I become 'manly' if I start lifting weights?
   No. Unless you dress up like a man and walk out of your
   gym, you won't look like one!

   On a serious note, most women don't have the same
   testosterone levels as men, and unless we have high levels
   of testosterone, we can't muscle up naturally. If you take
   steroids and supplements, then yes, chances are you will
   start to look beefier. But do this at your own risk: the side
   effects may be hazardous. At times, when we see a certain
   person looking heavy after they train, it is because training
   makes you hungry and if you are not eating in a calorie

deficit you will still be gaining weight while training. So, what you probably notice is not muscle gain, but fat gain.[3]

On the contrary, it will do the opposite for a woman: tighten and tone *all* over your body, burn fat, and shape your curves exactly how you want them to be. So, the next time you head to a gym, please don't restrict yourself to the treadmill and get to that strength-training room. You need not hesitate in picking up those barbells and dumb-bells (and make sure you have someone to spot you when you do this). You now know that it will not make you 'Bulky', 'Beefy', 'Manly' or a 'She-Hulk'.[4]

3. Won't lifting heavy weights lead to back problems and injuries?
    It's the other way around, actually. Lifting weights, under supervision, will prevent injuries, help your bones get stronger and cure your existing problems. That said, if you take up a membership at a gym somewhere, and go pick up a bar and start lifting heavy weights on your very first day, that would be a mistake and it will definitely have consequences. It is the same if you see a video on YouTube and start doing your own training without having any knowledge about how to pick up and drop your weights and engage the core while training and perform them without guidance. There's a right way of doing this, which involves a systematic progression from

[3] https://www.issaonline.com/blog/index.cfm/2016/ladies-lifting-heavy-wont-make-you-bulk-up.
[4] https://www.shape.com/fitness/tips/5-reasons-why-lifting-heavy-weights-wont-make-you-bulk.

body weight exercises to weights and then loads. You need to go to a good, certified professional, explain your problems and discuss your goals with them. Don't go overboard with weights without supervision.

4. I work out every day. Why am I still not losing the excess weight?

Because working out is only a small part of fat loss. You need to simultaneously be on a calorie-deficit. That is the most difficult and important part. You can kick-start your fat loss by merely focusing on your nutrition without even working out.

5. Will taking whey protein affect my kidneys?

No. Whey protein is nothing but a by-product that is processed and made into a concentrate while making cheese. It contributes to the protein that you need to perform, and to repair the muscle tear after your workout session. I haven't heard of anyone so far who has damaged their kidneys, liver or anything else as a result of consuming moderate amounts of whey protein.[5] But regardless of whether you have a kidney problem or not, consult your doctor before starting out, because they know you personally and can give the best advice.

For those of you who are lactose-intolerant, there is whey isolate where the lactose is removed to a large

---

[5] https://www.webmd.com/vitamins/ai/ingredientmono-833/whey-protein#:~:text=Whey%20protein%20is%20the%20protein,used%20as%20a%20protein%20supplement; https://blogs.ubc.ca/communicatingchemistry2017w110/2017/10/02/does-whey-protein-really-effect-kidney/.

extent. The fat is even further reduced, and it tastes less milky too. For vegans, soy protein and pea protein varieties are available.

6. Should I work out in the morning or in the evening?
   I have heard that Akshay Kumar wakes up at 4 a.m. every day and heads for his workout sessions. I have also heard that Salman Khan finishes up his entire day's work and his night shoots, and then hits the gym at 11 p.m. We see Dwayne Johnson sharing on social media how no matter which part of the world he is in, he finds a way to train without excuses. If you do not already follow him on Instagram, please do, for there were many days when I wouldn't feel up to it to get a session done, but seeing his determination to train hard at 3 a.m. after a long day of work would make me grab my water bottle and at least go for a run.

   Working out in the mornings helps me face the day with higher energy levels. Also, I don't have the niggling worry about squeezing in a pending gym session later in the day. When I wake up at 5 a.m., I feel like I'm fresh, wide awake, and ready to push myself to the maximum.

   But I know a few people who prefer to work out in the evenings after work, before they go to bed. They say that waking up early isn't feasible for them, and that the evenings are cooler. They also love the idea of finishing the day with a workout, going home and having a good meal after that, and then crashing to bed with a satisfying feeling of exhaustion.

   It really doesn't matter as long as you get it done!

7. Can I work out during my period?

    It really depends on a case by case basis. The side effects
    of periods vary from person to person. For some, it can
    be a painful set of days where your body deals with severe
    cramps and bloating—you definitely don't want to push
    your body even more on those days, so it's better to stay off
    heavy workouts. If you feel like getting some movement,
    you can maybe do something mild like walking or a nice
    long stretching session. As for me, I understand specifically
    how my cycle works each time and tweak my exercise
    regimen accordingly. I mostly do a nice walk on the heavy
    flow days and if I feel completely okay, I hit the gym.
    Doing some activity during my periods is a mood shifter
    for me and I instantly feel the serotonin and dopamine
    levels rising. At the end of the day, it is important to listen
    to what our body is telling us and following that while
    keeping things in balance.

8. Is it okay to have fruits in the night?

    Ayurvedic practices do not advocate the concept of having
    fruit in the night.

    My theory on this has already been explained in the
    earlier chapter about calories. Fruits, *phulkas*, rice or millets
    are all just different sources of carbs.

    I don't like the idea of fearing any type of food. When
    you eat and even how much you eat doesn't matter, as
    long as it is under the total amount of calories you should
    be consuming for yourself, if your goal is only addressing
    weight loss. But I personally build in the majority of my
    carb intake in and around my workouts, which is in the

morning for that's when I train. Why? So that the carb gets used up for energy and recovery and doesn't spike my insulin levels. Fruits can be treated as simple carbs and I would suggest you to follow the same thing that I do.

9.   What is good to have during and after a workout?
It depends on when you work out and how you feel. I generally have a snack, such as fruit—a banana, a green or red apple, or sometimes even a teaspoon of peanut butter—if I work out in the afternoon. Since fruits have fibre in them, unlike fruit juice, they are the healthier option.

When I want to start my workout right after waking up, I often drink a hot cup of black coffee and work out on an empty stomach. But on some days, if I feel hungry after waking up, I take an intra-workout blend of whey protein and fruit juice . . . I love it!

My post-workout meals usually comprise complex carbs—dal, *pesarattu*, sambar, overnight oats, eggs, millets, poha, soya, tofu, pulses, legumes, lentils, *kootu* and smoothies.

Part IV

Your Guidebook to Nutrition

27

How to Track Macros

Every few months, a fashionable term floats across all health and fitness platforms—a new yo-yo diet, a new exercise or a new trending fitness hashtag on social media. But one that has pretty much been consistent for a while now is calorie counting and eating according to your macronutrient requirements. This is also known as the Flexible Diet Plan or If It Fits Your Macros (IIFYM) plan.[1]

Counting macros and tracking my calories and macronutrients has been by far the most sensible way of eating for me. When I track my macros, I don't feel deprived of any single macronutrient while splurging on another. For example, if I have some chips with my lunch, by tracking it I know how much of my fat allowance is over, and that I need to start focusing on my veggies, carbs, and proteins for the remainder of the day.

---

[1] https://www.healthline.com/nutrition/iifym-guide#:~:text=IIFYM%
2C%20or%20%E2%80%9CIf%20It%20Fits,namely%20protein%2C%20
fat%20and%20carbohydrates.

I also don't have to resist foods that I feel tempted to eat (like a cup of tea with sugar and milk that helps me face the day or the weekend scoop of ice cream I like to sit with after lunch when I get that craving to have it). I log them in advance and understand my portions and eat accordingly. It is almost like a game where you have a daily allowance given— you lose points when you make the wrong choices, and you are rewarded with additional points to enjoy yourself with when you have done a good job of tracking and adjusting and manoeuvring without feeling deprived of anything.

To those of you who haven't been introduced to this yet, the 'macros eating' is a style of eating where you know and understand the amount of carbs, proteins and fats that your body needs.

What are macros?

'Macros' is an abbreviation of 'macronutrients'. Macronutrients are nutritional components in our diet that are needed in large amounts. These are mostly carbohydrates, fats and proteins.

To calculate your macros, it's a good idea to get some initial help from your trainer or nutritionist. Based on your sex, weight, height, daily activity, goals and other factors, you'll be given guidance on your total macros (i.e., calorie intake, carbs, fats, and proteins) and their daily allowances.

What You Need Before You Start

Even before I go any further, I would like to inform you that any product recommendations made here in this book are based on my own experiences and I am not promoting anything that I don't use myself not am I getting paid for any reference made to a particular person/brand/product/service/ website.

Buy a food scale for measurements if you don't have one already. Before you think that this will make you obsess over the amount of food you eat, let me clarify that this is not something you will do forever, and it is only for you to learn and get more accurate information about what you eat. A handful of rice can be different for different people based on the size of their palm, whereas when I say 30 g of rice, I am referring to only one measurement universally. That's why I want to reinforce this and say that you should weigh your food. A food scale is not expensive, and it will be very beneficial to you in the long run.

Also, download a food tracking application. There are lots of mobile applications on the AppStore or Play Store, but my personal favourite is MyFitnessPal, which has a free version as well as a paid version that you can pick. You can do everything that you need to on the free version itself. I like that it has a lot of features to track things with, a large database of different kinds of food, and that it is very user friendly. You can use other applications as well, based on your preferences.

General Steps Involved in Knowing Your Macros

Step 1: Track Your Normal Intake for One Full Week

I used to underestimate how much I ate, and overestimated how much I worked out until I was introduced to logging. Being aware of what and how much I was actually eating and where I was not eating substantially enough was an important step in this journey.

Be honest with yourself, and do not leave anything out. You do not need to get conscious at this point and change your regular eating habits when you start tracking. Getting you to feel guilty is not the intent. It is only to understand and get an accurate reflection of where you are in your journey and how much progress you are making. So log absolutely everything, from the extra helping of biriyani to the chocolate bar that you eat in between meals.

I even play a game where I estimate the serving size of something and then actually weigh it to see how close I was. It helped me learn a lot about portion sizes, which came in handy later on when I went to eat out at a friend's place or at a restaurant. Also, before you begin knowing your macros and do the actual logging, one week of normal logging helps you play around with the application you download and get used to it and figure things out. Use this time to learn and familiarize yourself with the process.

At the end of the full week, add each day's calories together and divide it by seven to find your average calorie intake per day.

I currently eat about _____ calories per day.

Though macro counting is something that can be applied to fat loss, maintenance and muscle gain, I am only taking fat loss into account here as it is the most popular one.

Step 2

To save yourself from all the calculations to arrive at your calorie needs, simply use this link:

https://www.calculator.net/macro-calculator.html.[2]

You need to choose the metric system, enter your age, gender, height, weight, and goal details, including how fast or slow you want to achieve your goal and sit back for the system to work out the math for you (which, however, is only an estimate).

Step 3

The results for different types of macro plans (low-fat, high-carb, high-protein, etc.) will be shown and you can choose any of those or stick to the balanced format, which is my preferred one too.

But as I said earlier, note that these calculations are not customized for Indian bodies and will, therefore, be exaggerated and need to be tweaked further. For this I cannot guide you in a generic manner in this book. For someone starting out in this journey, I suggest seeking a qualified nutritionist than trialling this out on yourself.

Step 4: Understand Your Macro Nutrients

Proteins: 4 calories/g
Fats: 9 calories/g
Carbs: 4 calories/g

Proteins are the most important macronutrient for me as I have personally seen the changes with and without adequate

---

[2] I am not in any way affiliated with this or any other website except my own brand Stay Fit with Ramya.

proteins both from a nutrition (protein makes me feel satiated for a long time) as well as a strength perspective (I tend to lift heavier, feel stronger and have leaner muscles too).

Carbohydrates are the body's preferred fuel source and are stored as glycogen when not used. Individuals who have physically demanding jobs work best on a high-carb diet, whereas for others, moderate carbs are ideal since their work is mostly sedentary and excess carbs only get stored as fat eventually.

Fats are important to regulate hormones, for vitamin absorption and for the brain to function.

Remember these before you start:

- No matter how perfect our macro goals are, if we don't track them right or can't hit them consistently, they will be useless.

- This is simply a guideline that I wanted to provide for you to understand how macro tracking works.

- Macros are not magical, and the whole process of 'macros eating' involves trial and error. That is perfectly normal. Ideally, take the help of an expert before you start, if possible, and also after you start when you struggle to make your own adjustments.

- If you have a medical condition or you are lactating or pregnant, it goes without saying that nothing should be done without expert supervision.

- If you find it overwhelming and hard to track all the macros at one go, just hitting your proteins and your calorie numbers when you start is a good stepping stone.

- You won't feel hungry when you are doing macro eating in the right way, including if you hit the fibre intake with boiled or raw fruits and vegetables. Also understand the exact hunger cues from your body, and don't get confused between thirst and hunger. If the desire to eat truly exists, increase your fibre intake and increase the volume of the vegetables you eat. In spite of all of this, if you still feel hungry, your macros probably need to be reworked again.

28

Why I Like Macro Eating the Most

The kind of flexibility that macro counting gives me particularly helps me keep track of things when there is a shift in my regular meal patterns. Whenever I travel somewhere where my options are limited, go to a friend's house, order in or dine out, I am always aware of what I'm eating and how much of it I can have, so I can then balance it out with my other meals. There are even days when I skip breakfast because I don't feel too hungry—that way, I save those calories and enjoy a good, wholesome meal for lunch instead.

To help you get started if you are new to this, here are some tips for effective macros tracking:

- Be disciplined. Track your macros each and every time you eat, without procrastinating.
- Don't enter false data. By providing false data, you will only cheat yourself.
- Remember, it is not just about weight loss but also about how you feel. For example, if you have a good amount

of fat allowance in your macro quotient and you decide to use all of it on a packet of French fries every day, you might meet your goal, but you'll neither feel good nor be healthy.

- Tracking your macros is better than depriving yourself of food you desperately crave and regretting it later on. It is also better than going overboard and feeling terribly guilty afterwards, then starving yourself as punishment for going off-track.

I love to hit my goals by tracking macros. Here are several reasons why I feel that this is effective.

I Can Make Sure I Am Getting Enough of All the Macronutrients

Earlier, I realized through all the diets I was experimenting with that I was still on a calorie deficit through my restricted eating, but was not meeting sufficient macros individually. This was not sustainable. We live in a world where women especially are always told to eat less, so these arbitrary numbers were widely floating around, and I started doing a 1200 calorie diet randomly because that was the popular calorie deficit number then. All that mattered to me was to cut my calories to that.

My metabolism was dipping down and was all over the place at that time. I was in a binge and restrict cycle because my calories were low and I was starving. It was a vicious cycle as I believed that the fewer calories I ate, the greater would be the fat loss. Honestly, this was just me being silly without understanding that fat loss is more about eating effectively and doing something that is sustainable and consistent.

I Become Aware of What I Eat

The problem I faced constantly with specific diets like intermittent fasting (IF) and keto when I followed them for a long time was that they were great when I started, but then I stopped seeing the results after a while and I didn't know what to do next. My clients would ask me the same. What to do when they plateau? That's why when I do something that requires quantifying, like macro eating, I can go ahead and make adjustments as necessary. This manipulation then helps me get the results I want, and it also helps me know how much and what I need to do next (for example, decrease my carbs a bit or balance between proteins and carbs).

The Focus Is More on Fat Loss and Not Weight Loss

When I consciously focus on meeting my macros and hitting my protein intake every day, I optimize on maintaining my muscle while being on a deficit. That, in turn, maximizes my fat loss and minimizes my muscle loss. I have learnt over the years that the more the muscle in my body, the more my metabolic rate increases too.[1] Thus, manipulating macros helps me burn fat more effectively.

---

[1] https://www.webmd.com/fitness-exercise/features/get-more-burn-from-your-workout#:~:text=When%20you%20increase%20your%20muscle,training%20to%20an%20exercise%20program.%22 (refer to tip 1).

I Practise Moderation

Eating healthy also needs to be worked on in a way that suits us. I have seen many clients who come to me saying that they are eating healthy and yet aren't able to reduce their body fat. I would then learn through pictures of their food that their portions of healthy food would be far too much. It is always an 'all or nothing' approach that we get caught up in when it comes to eating healthy. It's either junk food all the way, or avoiding flour and processed foods entirely, neither of which is ideal. Just like the 80/20 principle, macro eating allows me to specifically outline my fats, proteins, and carbohydrates. Thus, I can include food that I enjoy eating while knowing that I won't be able to hit my macros properly if the majority of my overall intake isn't coming from real and wholefoods. That's why I love macro eating, because it teaches me about the nutritional value of each food that I eat, the portions of food, and how to balance things properly so that I can eat without guilt and deprivation.

I don't believe that one needs to track macros for their entire life. I get to tracking only when I decide to go on a cut. While I am on maintenance, I take a more intuitive approach to eating. I also track my protein intake diligently, especially when I start calorie surplus eating to build muscle. But to get to that stage of intuitive eating, where I can simply estimate what food contains how much calories or know if it provides carbohydrates or proteins or fats, it took a long period of conscious tracking.

If you are convinced by this point, give it a shot after reaching out to an expert or come join me on Stay Fit With

Ramya (https://stayfitwithramya.exlyapp.com/) where we have a full team of certified and experienced nutritionists and personal trainers with me as a health coach to guide you.

But keep on reading for other tips!

I often see people complaining on social media that they are sick of tracking and that it drains them out. If you are sick of it and it's not serving you anymore, please stop doing it. It is that simple. Just like I may not want to do twenty hours of intermittent fasting, you may not enjoy this procedure—that is perfectly fine! There is always a cost associated in reaching a goal, and if that cost becomes too great for anyone, I think that it's okay to stop. The knowledge I get about nutrition and portions by tracking for a short period never leaves me, and that is why I love to do it. I do take breaks when I don't want to constantly track. I don't always rely on an app to tell me if I have enough proteins after I know what amount of protein my body needs and how to meet it.

What is important is being consistent, monitoring your progress and adjusting your numbers when and if needed. Whether I travel for work, take vacations to go to various places or even other special occasions, staying on top of macros has helped me maintain balance and follow a consistent plan without any struggles. Therefore, in my opinion, diving into macro counting is the best way to reach my fitness goals!

29

Recipes

I asked my friend Aruna Vijay to give us some fantastic, easy-to-make regional healthy recipes as she is very passionate and has a keen interest in food history and ingredients. Aruna is an entrepreneur, recipe developer and culinary enthusiast. She and I both believe that cooking is not just about learning new recipes, but more about integrating the right combination of ingredients, its cultural significance and the history of cuisines. We have together prepared a variety of recipes that you can check on my YouTube channel, Stay Fit With Ramya. Here are some of Aruna's delicious and nutrient-rich recipes that she has worked hard on just for you!

A few guidelines:[1]

* Vegetables should make up half of your plate. Aim for colours and variety on the plate.

---

[1] https://www.hsph.harvard.edu/nutritionsource/healthy-eating-plate/;
https://www.who.int/news-room/fact-sheets/detail/healthy-diet.

- Vegetables are very low in calories, though it depends on the preparation method—steaming and stir frying are better than deep frying. In addition, vegetables like potato are high in calories and need to be consumed in moderation. Proteins are very crucial when you workout. Check on your protein intake in each and every meal.

- Carbohydrates can be ideally planned after your workout to utilize them effectively for energy. Opt for non-refined whole grains such as brown rice, millets and oats; if your carbs include fruits, then opt for watery and local fruits that are low in sugar.

- Be mindful of your fats while cooking. Avoid trans-fat entirely, and go easy on saturated fats too.

- Restrict the intake of sugary soft drinks or avoid them altogether. Maintain good water intake to ensure optimal hydration.

- Eat home-cooked food and avoid eating out or ordering in as much as possible.

- Stay away from processed foods of any kind.

- Remember that you are what you eat, and abs are made in the kitchen.

HEALTH DRINKS

3-Spice Water

These three are the magical spices in Indian cooking. *Ajwain* helps to control gastritis, cumin helps in digestion, and fennel helps in controlling bloating.[2]

Ingredients

- Ajwain/Omum – 1 tsp
- Fennel seeds – 1 tsp
- Jeera/Cumin Seeds – 1 tsp
- Water – 2 cups

Procedure

- Mix all the ingredients and boil till the water reduces to half.
- Enjoy this warm.

Tips

- You can make a big batch of it and consume it the whole day.
- You could also make a powder of these spices and store it.
- You can have this during your intermittent fasting window.

---

[2] https://www.ncbi.nlm.nih.gov/pmc/articles/PMC4096002/; https://www.ncbi.nlm.nih.gov/pmc/articles/PMC4096002/; https://www.healthline.com/nutrition/9-benefits-of-cumin#TOC_TITLE_HDR_4.

Health Report

- Calories – 30
- Fats – 1.4 g
- Carbs – 3.9 g
- Proteins – 1 g

Banana Stem Juice

Ingredients

- Banana stem chopped – 1 cup
- Water – ½ cup
- Salt – a pinch

Procedure

- Grind banana stem and water
- Strain it and add salt
- Consume it immediately

Tips

- You need to discard the outer skin of the stem.
- After chopping, leave it in buttermilk to avoid discolouration.
- Drink it immediately.

Health Report

- Calories – 20
- Fats – 0.3 g

- Carbs – 3 g
- Proteins – 0.9 g

Golden Concoction

This helps in flushing out toxins during the day. It slows down the release of sugar and fat stored in cells.[3]

Ingredients

- Cinnamon powder – 1 tsp
- Water – 2 cups
- Grated ginger – ½ tsp
- Juice of half lemon

Procedure

- Boil water, cinnamon and ginger for 15 minutes.
- Strain it and add lemon juice.
- Enjoy it warm.

Tips

- You can make a big batch and consume it 5 times a day.
- Add lemon juice only while drinking it.

Health Report

- Calories – 8
- Fat – 0.3 g

---

[3] John Davidson, Health Benefits of Cinnamon (JD-Biz Corp Publishing, 2014).

- Carbs – 2.4 g
- Proteins – 0.1 g

Lemon Chia Water

This helps in flushing out toxins during the day. It slows down the release of sugar and fat stored in body cells.

Ingredients

- Warm water – 1 cup
- Chia seeds/sabja seeds – 1 tsp
- Lemon juice – 1 tsp
- Salt – a pinch

Procedure

- In a cup, add hot water and chia seeds and mix.
- Stir it for a few minutes for it to bloom and add lemon juice.
- Enjoy it warm.

Tips

- You could also do this with room temperature water.

Health Report

- Calories – 20
- Fats – 1.5 g

- Carbs – 1.3 g
- Proteins – 0.7 g

Mom's Night–Time Ritual

Ingredients

- Almonds – 5
- Poppy seeds – 1 tsp
- Sesame seeds – 1 tsp
- Black pepper – 3
- Saffron – a few strands (optional)
- Milk – ½ cup
- Turmeric – ¼ tsp

Procedure

- Soak everything for 5 hours or overnight (except milk) in half a cup of water.
- Add all the ingredients in a food processor except for milk and blend till smooth
- Then transfer the paste to a pan, add milk, turmeric and bring it to a boil.
- Serve it warm.

Tips

- Peel the almonds before grinding.

Health Report[4]

- Calories – 156
- Fats – 9.1 g
- Carbs – 12.3 g
- Proteins – 7.2 g

SNACKS

Cucumber Logs

A quick snack loaded with vitamins that will keep you full and hydrated.

Ingredients

- Native/small cucumber – 1
- Yogurt – 2 tsp
- Green chutney – 2 tsp
- Red chilli powder – 1 tsp
- Salt/chaat masala – ½ tsp

Procedure

- Slit the cucumber vertically.
- Scoop out the seeds from the centre with the help of a spoon.
- Fill it with yogurt and remaining ingredients.
- Enjoy it fresh.

[4] Per cent daily values are based on a 2000 calories diet. Your daily value may be higher or lower depending on your calorie needs.

Tips

- The cucumber can be replaced with bell peppers.
- Yogurt could be replaced with crumbled paneer or hummus.
- You can play with flavours by changing the sauce and seasoning.
- Crushed peanuts can be added for crunch.

Health Report

- Calories – 79
- Fats – 2 g
- Carbs – 9.1 g
- Proteins – 4.1 g

Peanut Butter Apples

Peanut butter with apples is a classic combination.

Ingredients

- Thinly sliced apples – 1 cup
- Peanut butter or almond butter – 1 tsp
- Cinnamon powder – ¼ tsp
- Roasted nuts and seeds – 1 tsp

Procedure

- Cut and thinly slice the apples and arrange on a plate.

- Drizzle some peanut butter on the apples.
- Garnish with some roasted seeds and nuts.

Tips

- Apples tend to oxidize, so consume it immediately.
- If you are allergic to nuts, you could use melted dark chocolate.
- Make your own peanut butter to keep count of calories.

Health Report

- Calories – 158
- Fats – 11.3 g
- Carbs – 15.1 g
- Proteins – 5.6 g

Spicy Cream Cheese Dip

A spicy dip to enjoy your favourite veggies.

Ingredients

This portion makes 4 wraps.
- Paneer – ½ cup
- Hung curd – 2 tsp
- Water – 2 tsp
- Spicy Green Chutney – 2 tsp
- Thinly sliced veggies, tindora, cucumber, bell pepper, cabbage leaves – 5

Procedure

- In a food processor, add paneer, hung curd, chutney and water.
- Blend this into a smooth paste and adjust consistency.
- Take a cabbage leaf, add a spoonful of cream cheese.
- Layer the veggies and wrap it.

Tips

- You could also use hummus instead of cream cheese.
- Chill these wraps before serving for best results.

Health Report

Each wrap contains
- Calories – 60
- Fats – 2 g
- Carbs – 2.2 g
- Proteins – 4.6 g

Curry Leaf Granola

A crunchy snack with a desi twist.

Ingredients

This makes 12 tsp granola
- Torn curry leaves – ½ cup
- Rolled oats – 3 tsp

- Chopped almonds – 1 tsp
- Raisins – 1 tsp
- Chopped walnuts – 1 tsp
- Sambar masala – 1 tsp
- Pumpkin seeds – 1 tsp
- Oil – 1 tsp
- Salt – ½ tsp

Procedure

- In a bowl, mix oil and sambar masala, and add all the ingredients.
- Coat everything well with the masala.
- In a flat pan, roast this on the lowest flame till it's crunchy.
- Cool and store it in an airtight container.

Tips

- You could use any nuts and seeds of your choice.
- Make sure to roast on slow flame, tossing continuously.

Health Report

2 tsp of granola contains
- Calories – 75
- Fats – 5.2 g
- Carbs – 4.3 g
- Proteins – 2.3 g

Pottukadalai Laddoo

Ingredients

This recipe makes 5 bite-sized laddoos
- Pottukadalai – 3 tsp
- Almonds – 5
- Melted ghee – 1 tsp
- Jaggery powder – 1 tsp
- Sesame seeds – 1 tsp

Procedure

- In a pan, dry-roast almonds, pottukadalai and sesame seeds separately.
- In a small mixer jar, add the pottukadalai and make a powder.
- Remove it and add almonds and sesame seeds, then make coarse powder.
- Add all this to a plate, add hot melted ghee and jaggery powder and make small laddoos.

Tip

- You can add any nuts of your choice.

Health Report

Each laddoo contains
- Calories – 64

- Fats – 4 g
- Carbs – 7 g
- Proteins – 2 g

SOUPS AND COOLERS

Keerai Thandu Soup

Generally, the leaves of the keerai or amaranth are used and the stems are thrown away. But the stems have a lot of nutrients in them which are lost in the process.

Ingredients

- Keerai stem – 1 cup
- Chopped tomatoes – ½ cup
- Water – 2 cups
- Salt – 1 tsp
- Pepper – ½ tsp
- Turmeric – ¼ tsp

Procedure

- Chop and add all the ingredients (except pepper) in a pan and boil for 20 minutes.
- While it's still warm, mash it with your hands and strain it.
- Add pepper and boil again.
- Serve warm.

Tips

- If you don't have the stems you could also use the leaves.
- While boiling again you can also add some finely chopped veggies and add some more water if required.

Health Report

- Calories – 29
- Fats – 0.2 g
- Carbs – 5.8 g
- Proteins – 1 g

Homemade Protein Lemonade

Ingredients

- Roasted channa powder (Uppu kadalai) – 2 tsp
- Juice of half a Lemon
- Black salt – 1 tsp
- Few mint leaves
- Black pepper – ¼ tsp
- Sweetener – optional
- Water – ½ cup
- Ice cubes – 5

Procedure

- Add all the ingredients in a food processor and blend till smooth.
- Serve it fresh.

Tips

- You can add sugar if your diet allows it.
- Uppu kadalai is also called roasted yellow gram.

Health Report

- Calories – 140
- Fats – 1.7 g
- Carbs – 21 g
- Proteins – 7 g

Green Virgin Soup

A hearty green soup that you can include in your everyday diet.

Ingredients

- Chopped spinach – 1 cup
- Peas – ¼ cup
- Salt – 1 tsp
- Pepper – ½ tsp
- Milk – ¼ cup
- Water – ½ cup
- Oliver oil – 1 tsp

Procedure

- In a pan add olive oil and sauté peas for a couple of minutes.
- Then add spinach and cook till it wilts.

- Add water cover and cook for 10 minutes.
- Cool and puree it. Transfer it back to the pan and add milk, salt and pepper.
- Bring it to a boil and serve warm.

Tip

- Zucchini can be used instead of green peas.

Health Report

- Calories – 113
- Fats – 6.6 g
- Carbs – 9.2 g
- Proteins – 4.9 g

Creamy Bottle Gourd Soup

This is an excellent low-calorie soup; it is also filling and nutritious.

Ingredients

- Chopped bottle gourd – 1 cup
- Soaked and peeled almonds – 5 pcs
- Onion – ¼ cup
- Olive oil – 1 tsp
- Salt – ½ tsp
- Pepper – ¼ tsp

Procedure

- In a cooker, add oil and sauté the bottle gourd and onion.
- Then add water, soaked almonds and salt and pressure cook for 2 whistles.
- Cool and puree it.
- Then add corn flour with 2 tsp water and add it to the puree.
- Add milk to adjust the consistency.
- Reheat and serve warm.
- Add some roasted sliced almonds for garnish.

Tip

- Peel the almonds before cooking.

Health Report

- Calories – 130
- Fats – 6.8 g
- Carbs – 10 g
- Proteins – 4 g

Moringa Lentil Soup

Moringa is becoming known to the world as the new superfood.

Ingredients

- Chopped drumsticks – 1 cup
- Soaked toor dal – 1 tsp
- Salt – ½ tsp
- Water – 1 cup
- Pepper – ¼ tsp
- Juice of half a lime
- Chopped cilantro

Procedure

- In a pressure cooker add chopped drumsticks, dal, salt, water and pressure cook for 4 whistles.
- Release pressure naturally, let it cool down.
- Mash with hands and strain the pulp.
- Warm again, serve with juice of half a lime, pepper and chopped cilantro.

Tip

- You can also use yellow dal.

Health Report

- Calories – 150
- Fats – 5 g
- Carbs – 11 g
- Proteins – 14 g

Cucumber Coolant

On a busy day, when you don't have time to cook something healthy, this soup comes in handy, as you can prepare it in 10 minutes.

Ingredients

- Cucumber small – 2
- Coriander leaves – ½ cup
- Garlic – 1 clove
- Onion – 2 tsp
- Salt
- Pepper
- Hung yogurt – ¼ cup
- Spinach – a few leaves
- Green chilli – a small piece

Procedure

- Add everything in a food processor and blend till smooth.
- Transfer it to a bowl and cool it for a couple of hours before serving.
- Serve cold.

Tip

- Yogurt can be replaced with coconut milk.

Health Report

- Calories – 77
- Fats – 3 g
- Carbs – 8 g
- Proteins – 5 g

SALADS

Grilled Paneer Salad

Ingredients

- Paneer slice – 1 (50 g)
- Steamed green beans – handful
- Oil – 1 tsp
- Pinch of salt
- Sesame seeds – 1 tsp

Dressing:

- Oil – ½ tsp
- Finely chopped ginger garlic – 1 tsp
- Chilli sauce / Sriracha sauce – 1 tsp
- Tomato sauce – 1 tsp
- Soy sauce – 2 tsp

Procedure

- In a non-stick pan, add 1 tsp oil and cook the paneer on both sides with a pinch of salt till it's golden brown.

- Remove the paneer, and in the same pan stir-fry the steamed beans.
- In another pan, add oil and sauté the ginger garlic paste.
- Then, add all the sauces and a little water to adjust the consistency.
- Take a plate and place the paneer and beans on it.
- Pour the sauce over it.
- Enjoy it hot.

Tips

- You can use tofu if you are vegan or even use grilled cauliflower.
- Be mindful that paneer has fat too, so this can be served as a complete meal.

Health Report

- Calories – 292
- Fats – 19 g
- Carbs – 17.6 g
- Proteins – 13.8 g

Crunchy Cucumber Salad

Peanuts and cucumber are a match made in heaven. The softness of the cucumbers and the crunchiness of the peanuts are an amazing combination.

Ingredients

- Cucumber cubed – 1 cup
- Boiled black channa – ¼ cup
- Grated coconut – 1 tsp
- Green chilli – 1 small
- Crushed peanuts – 2 tsp
- Salt – ½ tsp
- Finely chopped coriander – ¼ cup
- Finely chopped raw mango – 2 tsp

Tempering:

- Coconut oil – 1 tsp
- Mustard seeds – 1 tsp
- Curry leaves – few

Procedure

- In a bowl, mix all the ingredients well, except for the tempered mixture.
- Take a pan, heat the oil, splutter mustard seeds and curry leaves.
- Pour the tempered mixture over the salad and enjoy it fresh.

Tips

- Instead of black channa you could use white channa, rajma or another sort of protein.
- Dry roast the peanuts before crushing it.

Health Report

- Calories – 260
- Fats – 15 g
- Carbs – 19.5 g
- Proteins – 5.1 g

Fridge-clearing Salad

On the days when you are unsure of what to eat, this salad is your go-to.

Ingredients

- Tomato chopped – ¼ cup
- Cucumber chopped – ¼ cup
- Chopped bell pepper – ¼ cup
- Chopped cabbage – ¼ cup
- Chopped pineapple – ¼ cup
- Pomegranate – ¼ cup
- Finely chopped coriander, mint, dill, baby spinach – ½ cup

Dressing:

- Olive oil – 1 tsp
- Salt – ½ tsp
- Pepper – ½ tsp
- Lime juice – 1 tsp

Procedure

- In a bowl, mix all the ingredients well, except for the dressing.
- Take a jar and add all the ingredients for the dressing and shake well.
- Pour this dressing over the salad and enjoy it fresh.

Tips

- You can use any veggies or fruits of your choice, but make sure to add a fruit for sweetness.
- Use loads of greens.

Health Report

- Calories – 194
- Fats – 14.4 g
- Carbs – 16.5 g
- Proteins – 2.3 g

Citrusy Salad

A sweet, tangy salad.

Ingredients

- Segmented Orange – ¾ cup
- Segmented Sweet lime – ¾ cup
- Coriander leaves chopped – ¼ cup

- Bean sprouts – ¼ cup
- Crushed peanuts – 2 tsp

Dressing:

- Garlic chopped – 1 tsp
- Green chilli – 1 small
- Tamarind pulp – 1 tsp
- Soy sauce – ½ tsp
- Jaggery – 1 tsp

Procedure

- In a bowl, add fruits, bean, sprouts, coriander and mix well.
- Take a mortar and pestle and add all the ingredients for the dressing and ground them.
- Pour this dressing over the salad and enjoy it fresh.
- Finally, add the crushed peanuts.

Tip

- You could also add in some crumbled goat's milk cheese.

Health Report

- Calories – 217
- Fats – 5.5 g
- Carbs – 35 g
- Proteins – 5.4 g

Protein Salad

Ingredients

- Cooked kabuli channa – ¼ cup
- Bean sprouts – ¼ cup
- Cubed paneer – ¼ cup
- Cooked kidney beans – ¼ cup
- Grated carrot – ¼ cup
- Finely chopped bell pepper – ¼ cup
- Juice of half lime
- Black salt – ½ tsp
- Cumin powder – 1 tsp

Procedure

- In a bowl, mix all the ingredients well.
- Adjust the seasoning according to your taste.

Tips

- Sprouted beans have more protein than regular ones.
- Cook the paneer on a pan till golden, if you don't like the raw taste of it.
- Be mindful that kidney beans contain carbs and can cause flatulence.

Health Report

- Calories – 242
- Fats – 10.6 g

- Carbs – 25.3 g
- Proteins – 11.8 g

Popeye Salad

Ingredients

- Spinach/keerai washed and finely chopped – 2 cups
- Dry red chilli – 1
- Mustard seeds – 1 tsp
- Curry leaves – a few
- Oil – 1 tsp
- Soaked yellow dal – 1 tsp
- Grated coconut – 1 tsp
- Salt – ½ tsp

Procedure

- In a pan add 1 tsp oil, mustard seeds, curry leaves, dry red chilli.
- Sauté it and add the greens, cover and cook.
- Halfway through, add the soaked dal and cover.
- Add salt and grated coconut and mix well.
- Enjoy this fresh.

Health Report

- Calories – 115
- Fats – 7.7 g
- Carbs – 7.7 g
- Proteins – 4.7 g

Kovakkai Salad

Ingredients

- Young tindora thinly sliced – 1 cup
- Thinly sliced bell peppers – ½ cup
- Thinly sliced green beans – ½ cup
- Salt – ½ tsp
- Oil – 1 tsp
- Grated coconut – 1 tsp
- Mustard seeds
- Dry red chilli – 2

Procedure

- In a pan, add 1 tsp oil, mustard seeds, curry leaves and dry red chilli.
- Sauté it and add the kovakkai, then add the remaining greens, cover and cook.
- Add salt and grated coconut and mix well.
- Enjoy this fresh.

Tips

- After cooking, the quantity will reduce to 1 cup.
- Coconut is optional, but it gives a nice aroma.
- You could use any greens of your choice.

Health Report

- Calories – 110
- Fats – 8 g
- Carbs – 9.4 g
- Proteins – 2.1 g

BREAKFAST

Papaya Chia Boat

Ingredients

- Small Papaya – cut vertically and deseeded
- Oats – 1 tsp
- Chia seeds – 1 tsp
- Regular milk – ½ cup
- Seeds and nuts – 1 tsp (optional)

Procedure

- In a bowl, combine oats, chia seeds and milk.
- Let this sit overnight in the fridge; you can adjust the consistency by adding a little water.
- While serving, scoop the papaya from the centre and remove seeds, then fill it with the overnight-soaked oats and chia.
- Sprinkle nuts and seeds.

Tips

- If you don't like combining chia and oats, you can use them separately.
- The same thing can be made in jar and topped with fruits.
- They can be made in advance and used over a couple of days.
- You can add cocoa to make it chocolate flavoured.

Health Report

- Calories – 228
- Fats – 8 g
- Carbs – 31 g
- Proteins – 9 g

Madras Uttapam

Ingredients

- Grated carrot – ¼ cup
- Finely chopped onion – ¼ cup
- Finely chopped bell pepper – ¼ cup
- Finely chopped cabbage – ¼ cup
- Green chilli – 1
- Finely chopped coriander – ¼ cup
- Chickpea flour – ¼ cup
- Salt
- Chilli powder – 1 tsp
- Ajwain – ½ tsp

- Water – ¼ cup (do not add all at once)
- Oil – 1 tsp

Procedure

- Mix all the ingredients and make a thick batter.
- Grease the pan and pour a small ladle of batter and cook on both sides.

Tips

- You can add any veggies of your choice.
- You can also add your daily dose of protein powder to it.

Health Report

- Calories – 169
- Fats – 6.2 g
- Carbs – 22.8 g
- Proteins – 6.5 g

When Banana Met Coffee

Banana and coffee are a match made in heaven. What better way to start your mornings than with this combination?

Ingredients

- Ripe banana – 1 small
- Instant coffee powder – 1 tsp

- Wheat flour – ½ cup
- Protein powder – 1 tsp (optional)
- Pinch of salt
- Baking soda – ½ cup
- Milk – approximately ¼ cup

Procedure

- In a food processor, add everything except baking soda and combine well.
- Transfer it to a bowl and add baking soda.
- Pour into a non-stick pan.
- Flip over after a couple of minutes and cook till golden brown.

Tips

- If you don't like coffee, you can substitute it for cocoa or skip it completely.
- Grease the pan if you are not using a non-stick pan.
- Add the baking soda just before pouring the batter.
- The batter should be slightly thick.

Health Report

- Calories – 204
- Fats – 1.5 g
- Carbs – 41 g
- Proteins – 6 g

'Sinlicious' Hot Chocolate

Ingredients

- Regular milk – 1 cup
- Unsweetened cocoa powder – 1 tsp
- Coffee granules – ¼ tsp (optional)
- Dark chocolate chips – 2 tsp
- Cinnamon powder – ¼ tsp (optional)

Procedure

- In a pan, warm the milk and add all the ingredients except for chocolate chips.
- Once the milk starts to become hot, remove from heat.
- Add the chocolate chips and stir till melted, then heat it again.
- Pour into a cup and enjoy it hot.

Tips

- If you don't like coffee, you can skip it completely.
- If you don't have chocolates chips, increase the quantity of cocoa powder.

Health Report

- Calories – 250
- Fats – 11.6 g
- Carbs – 26.8 g
- Proteins – 10.9 g

Green Goodness

Ingredients

- Amla – 1
- Cucumber – 1 small
- Spinach – a handful
- Coriander – ¼ cup
- Mint – ¼ cup
- Ginger – 1 inch
- Apple – half piece

Procedure

- Add all the ingredients in a food processor and blend till smooth.
- Serve it fresh.

Tips

- You can add ingredients based on availability.
- Daily dose of protein powder can be added to it.

Health Report

- Calories – 99
- Fats – 0.7 g
- Carbs – 22.8 g
- Proteins – 2.7 g

Skinny Cappuccino

Ingredients

- Regular milk – 1 cup
- Coffee granules – 2 tsp
- Unsweetened cocoa powder – 1 tsp
- Sweetener of your choice
- Ice cubes – 1 cup

Procedure

- Add all the ingredients in a food processor and blend till smooth.
- Serve it fresh.

Tips

- You can add sugar if your diet allows it.
- You can add any milk of your choice.

Health Report

- Calories – 150
- Fats – 5.5 g
- Carbs – 15 g
- Proteins – 9 g

FERMENTED FOOD

Beans Sprouts

Ingredients

- Green moong dal – 1 cup
- Water – ½ cup

Procedure

- Soak the dal overnight.
- Place the soaked beans on a damp cheesecloth or into a colander, and place that in a bowl.
- Cover the bowl.
- Keep the seeds in the dark, because the seeds get bitter when they come in contact with light.
- Keep sprinkling it with some water every couple of hours.
- By day 2, you will start noticing them sprout, so keep sprinkling water.
- By day 3, it should be ready, and you can store it in the fridge.

Health Report

- Calories – 159
- Fats – 0.6 g
- Carbs – 28.9 g
- Proteins – 10.8 g

Indian Sauerkraut

Ingredients

- Cabbage – 1 kg
- Carrot – 200 g
- Salt – 2 tsp
- Turmeric – 1 tsp
- Chilli powder – 1 tsp

Procedure

- In a wide bowl, add thinly sliced (1/2 inch thick) cabbage leaves, sliced carrot and salt.
- Massage it for 10 minutes with your hands, this will help the cabbage to wilt.
- Finally add in turmeric and chilli powder and mix well.
- Transfer this to a glass jar and press it down.
- Make sure the cabbage is tightly packed, so that it soaks in its own water.
- Place a cabbage leaf over the sauerkraut, cover the jar with a muslin cloth and put a rubber band to secure it.
- Close the lid loosely and keep it in a dark place for 5–6 days.
- Open and mix it well and transfer it to the fridge.

Tips

- Make sure there is enough empty space on top of the jar for the cabbage to ferment.

- When you open this for the first time, there could be a very strong smell, which is absolutely normal.
- Once open, refrigerate it and use it within 4–6 weeks.
- Use only a glass jar.

Health Report

Per serving of ¼ cup:
- Calories – 7
- Fats – 0.05 g
- Carbs – 1.52 g
- Proteins – 0.32 g

Fermented Pickle

Ingredients

- Carrot – ½ cup
- Cauliflower florets – ½ cup
- Pink salt – 2 tsp
- Ginger – 2 inch
- Green chilli – 2, slit
- Bay leaf – 4
- Water – 2 cups

Procedure

- In a sterilized glass jar, add the chopped vegetables, green chilli, ginger and bay leaf.

- In a separate bowl, add water, salt and mix well.
- Pour this in the jar over the vegetables and press the vegetables.
- The vegetables should be submerged in this brine, so leave some space on the top of the jar for it to ferment.
- Place a bay leaf on the top of the jar and cover it tightly, then keep it in a warm place for 4–5 days.
- Open the jar once every day, as it will let the air out, and you will see bubbles forming on the top.
- After 5 days, store this in the refrigerator.

Tips

- Make sure there is enough empty space on the top of the jar for it to ferment.
- When you open this for first time, there could be a very strong smell, which is absolutely normal.
- Once open, refrigerate it and use it within 4–6 weeks.

Health Report

Per 50 g it contains:
- Calories – 10
- Fats – 0 g
- Carbs – 2 g
- Proteins – 0 g

Indian Kombucha

Ingredients

- Carrot – 2 cups (cut like fries)
- Beetroot – 1 cup
- Yellow mustard – 1 ½ tsp
- Black salt – 1 ½ tsp
- Black pepper – 1 tsp
- Bay leaf – 1
- Water – 6 to 7 cups

Procedure

- Using a mortar and pestle, grind mustard and pepper into a coarse powder.
- Take a glass jar and add all the ingredients and mix well.
- Cover it with a muslin cloth and secure it with a rubber band.
- Do not close the jar tightly.
- Keep it near your kitchen window and let it ferment for 5–6 days.
- Keep stirring it once a day; the time taken for it to ferment depends on the climatic condition in your area.
- Once it's done, strain and transfer to another jar and keep the pickled veggies separately.
- It will have a sour, pungent and salty taste.
- Refrigerate and consume small quantities of it during lunch time.

Tips

- Make sure there is enough empty space on the top of the jar for it to ferment.
- When you open this for first time, there could be a very strong smell, which is absolutely normal.
- Once open, refrigerate it and use it within 4–6 weeks.

Health Report

- Calories – 40
- Fats – 1 g
- Carbs – 9 g
- Proteins – 1 g

MAIN COURSE

Cauliflower Curd Rice

No meal is complete without a bowl of curd rice.

Ingredients

- Grated cauliflower – ½ cup
- Grated ginger – 2 tsp
- Curd – ½ cup
- Milk – ¼ cup
- Salt – ½ tsp

Tempering:

- Curry leaves – a few
- Mustard seeds – 1 tsp
- Urad dal – ½ tsp
- Green chilli – 1 slit
- Oil – 1 tsp

Procedure

- In a bowl, add grated cauliflower, ginger, rice, curd, milk and salt.
- In a pan, heat oil, mustard seeds, urad dal, curry leaves and green chilli.
- Add the tempered mixture to the cauliflower curd rice and mix well.
- Let it cool down in the fridge for an hour before serving.

Health Report

- Calories – 180
- Fats – 9.8 g
- Carbs – 14 g
- Proteins – 9.2 g

Cabbage Kootu

Ingredients

To pressure cook:
- Cabbage chopped – 2 cups

- Soaked yellow dal – 3 tsp
- Onion finely chopped – ¼ cup
- Green chilli – 1 slit
- Sambar masala – 1 tsp
- Salt
- Water – ½ cup

Tempering:

- Curry leaves – a few
- Mustard seeds – 1 tsp
- Urad dal – ½ tsp
- Oil – 1 tsp

To grind:

- Grated coconut – 2 tsp
- Jeera – 1 tsp
- Green chilli – 1

Procedure

- In a cooker, add all the ingredients (except the tempered mixture) and pressure cook for 3 whistles on medium flame.
- Let the pressure release and open and mash it well, then add in the grounded paste.
- In a pan, heat oil, mustard seeds, urad dal, curry leaves and add the spinach mix.
- Serve warm.

Tip

- You can add any vegetables of your choice.

Health Report

- Calories – 180
- Fats – 9.8 g
- Carbs – 14 g
- Proteins – 9.2 g

Brinjal Curry

It's also called rasavangi, a mix between sambar and *kootu*.

Ingredients

- Brinjal – 1 cup
- Tamarind water – ½ cup
- Water – ½ cup
- Cooked toor dal – ¼ cup
- Salt – 1 tsp
- Turmeric powder

Curry *podi*:

- Oil – 1 tsp
- Channa dal – 1 tsp
- Coriander seeds – 2 tsp
- Dry red chilli – 3

- Grated coconut – 2 tsp
- Rice – 1 tsp

Tempering:

- Oil – 1 tsp
- Mustard seeds – 1 tsp
- Curry leaves – 1 few
- Asafoetida – ¼ tsp

Procedure

- Cook the toor dal and keep it aside.
- In a pan, add the brinjal, water, salt, turmeric and bring it to a boil; when the brinjal is half-done, add in the tamarind water and cook till soft.
- In a pan, add oil, channa dal, coriander seeds, rice and red chilli. Cook till the dal is brown, for a couple of minutes. Switch off the gas, add in the grated coconut and sauté it in the retained heat. Cook and grind to a fine powder.
- Once the brinjal is cooked, add the ground curry powder and cooked dal and mix well.
- Finally, heat oil, mustard seeds, curry leaves and asafoetida and pour this over the brinjal.

Tip

- The curry should be slightly thick; adjust the spice level according to your taste.

Health Report

- Calories – 18
- Fats – 9.8 g
- Carbs – 14 g
- Proteins – 9.2 g

Aviyal

Ingredients

- Water – ¼ cup
  Length-wise chopped veggies (drumsticks, French beans, podlanga, white pumpkin) – 1 ½ cup

  To grind into a fine paste:

- Coconut – ¼ cup
- Small onion – 2
- Green chilli – 1
- Cumin – ½ tsp
- Curd – ¼ cup
- Salt – 1 tsp

  Tempering:

- Coconut oil – 1 tsp
- Mustard seeds – ½ tsp
- Curry leaves - few

Procedure

- Add the vegetables, salt and water and pressure cook for 1 whistle.
- Switch off the flame immediately and let the pressure settle.
- Open and check if the veggies are soft, then add in the ground paste carefully, without breaking the vegetables.
- Cook for a couple of minutes more, switch off the gas and add in the curd, then mix it well.
- Finally pour the tempering.

Tip

- The curry should be slightly thick; adjust the spice level according to your taste.

Health Report

- Calories – 220
- Fats – 13 g
- Carbs – 18.4 g
- Proteins – 6.8 g

Curry Leaf Thogayal

Thogayal is basically a type of chutney. Curry leaves are great for hair and skin issues, and it also has many medicinal properties. This is a great way to add it to your diet.

Ingredients

- Curry leaves – 2 cups
- Coriander leaves – 1 cup
- Urad dal – 1 tsp
- Channa dal – 1 tsp
- Dry red chilli – 7 to 8
- Nelika/Gooseberry –1
- Asafoetida – 1 tsp
- Salt to taste
- Oil – 1 tsp
- Water – 2 to 3 tsp

Procedure

- In a pan, add oil, sauté the dal till golden brown.
- Then add the dry chilli, tamarind and asafoetida.
- Finally, add in the curry leaves and coriander. Then, just sauté for couple of seconds and switch off the heat and cook in the retained heat.
- Add salt and grind to a coarse, thick paste; add water only if required.

Tip

- This can be stored in the fridge for 4–5 days.

Health Report

- Calories – 140
- Fats – 6.6 g

- Carbs – 45.1 g
- Proteins – 6.8 g

Spicy Green Chutney

Ingredients

- Coriander leaves – 2 cups
- Mint leaves – 1 cup
- Green chilli – 3
- Garlic – 2 cloves
- Lemon juice – 1 tsp
- Cumin seeds – 1 tsp
- Salt – 1 tsp
- Sugar – a pinch
- Ice cubes – 5

Procedure

- Grind everything in a mixer jar to a smooth chutney.
- Store in fridge for a week.

Health Report

- Calories – 207
- Fats – 0.3 g
- Carbs – 38.1 g
- Proteins – 4.5 g

Okra Podi Curry

Ingredients

- Oil – 1 tsp
- Okra chopped – 1 cup
- Turmeric powder – ¼ tsp
- Salt to taste
- Curry leaves
- Asafoetida – ¼ tsp

To grind podi:

- Oil – 1 tsp
- Coriander seeds – 2 tsp
- Channa dal – 1 tsp
- Urad dal – 1 tsp
- Sesame seeds – ½ tsp
- Dry red chilli – 3

Procedure

- In a pan, add oil, sauté all the ingredients, then grind and cook and make a coarse powder.
- In a pan, add 1 tsp oil, asafoetida, curry leaves and add the okra, salt and turmeric.
- Sauté for couple of minutes and cover and cook for 4–5 minutes.
- Stir once in between. Once the okra is soft, add the *podi* and cook for a few minutes. Switch off the heat.

Tip

- The podi can be made and stored in advance and used for any vegetables.

Health Report

- Calories – 140
- Fats – 6.6 g
- Carbs – 45.1 g
- Proteins – 6.8 g

Vazhaipoo Thoran

Vazhaipoo (banana flower) is loaded with health benefits.

Ingredients

- Banana flower chopped – 1 cup
- Onion finely chopped – ¼ cup
- Cooked black channa – 2 tsp
- Salt to taste
- Oil – 1 tsp
- Mustard seeds – 1 tsp
- Curry leaves – a few
- Dry red chilli – 2
- Grated coconut – 2 tsp

Procedure

- First clean the banana flower by removing the outer cover.
- Chop it finely and soak it in thin butter milk or vinegar water to avoid oxidation.
- Steam the banana stem to soften it.
- In a pan, add oil and mustard seeds, and let it splutter.
- Add curry leaves, dry red chillies and onions. Cook till the onions turn pink.
- Add the steamed banana flower, cooked black channa and cook for a couple of minutes.
- Finally, add salt and grated coconut.

Tip

- Add salt in the last step.

Health Report

- Calories – 142
- Fats – 7.5 g
- Carbs – 16.1 g
- Proteins – 3 g

DESSERT

Chocolate Barks

Ingredients

- Dark chocolates chips – ½ cup (70 per cent cocoa)
- Chopped almonds – 2 tsp

Procedure

- Take a deep pan and fill half of it with water.
- Keep a wide bowl on it, as the water should not touch the bowl.
- Add the ¼ cup of chocolate to the bowl, keep the flame on medium and melt it.
- Take it off the flame and add in the remaining chocolate and whisk in the retained heat.
- Once the chocolate melts completely, pour it on parchment paper and spread it thin.
- Add the chopped nuts and keep it in the fridge for it to set.
- Once it sets, break it and enjoy.

Tips

- You can melt the chocolate in a microwave.
- Place it in the microwave and cook it for 10 seconds, take it out and stir, and repeat till it's done.

Health Report

- Calories – 211
- Fats – 13.7 g
- Carbs – 27 g
- Proteins – 3.1 g

Frozen Yoghurt Things

Ingredients

- Yoghurt – ½ cup
- Honey – 1 tsp
- Chia seeds – 1 tsp
- Pomegranate seeds – 1 tsp

Procedure

- Take yoghurt in a bowl, add honey and whisk till it's smooth.
- Pour it over parchment paper and spread it.
- Sprinkle chia seeds and pomegranate and freeze it.
- Break it and enjoy.

Tips

- Make sure your yoghurt is not sour and the consistency is thick.
- Use Greek yoghurt if possible.
- You can add any fruits of your choice.
- Honey is optional.

Health Report

- Calories – 146
- Fats – 6 g

- Carbs – 13.9 g
- Proteins – 10.8 g

Oats Payasam

A super quick dessert to fulfil your cravings for sweets.

Ingredients

- Oats – 3 tsp
- Milk – ½ cup
- Ghee – ½ tsp
- Cardamom powder – 1/8 tsp
- Saffron – few
- Jaggery powder – 1 ½ tsp

Procedure

- In a pan, add ghee and roast oats till slightly brown.
- Add milk and boil it over a slow flame.
- Once the milk has boiled and the oats have softened, add cardamom and saffron.
- Finally, add jaggery after switching off the gas.

Tips

- Use roasted oats.
- Switch off the gas before adding jaggery, as the milk may curdle.

Health Report

- Calories – 202 g
- Fats – 5.5 g
- Carbs – 31 g
- Proteins – 4.6 g

Part V

Mind Your Mind

30

When I Hit Rock Bottom

I used to be the kind of person who craved outside approval for every aspect of my life. I think it came about from the time I chose a career that was not what my parents had thought for me. They may have probably wanted me to pursue a regular engineering degree, do a job for a year or two, get married and be 'settled' before 25. They have completely supported me in all the decisions for my own happiness and have stood by me, but I am not too sure if they were happy about the decisions I'd made. I think this was deeply rooted in me, and so for some reason I always craved external validation and approval from them and everyone around me in everything I did, from my everyday job of whether to do a certain assignment or not, to the choices in life like whom to marry or if I can go on a day trip with my friends, etc. I felt guilty that I didn't live up to their expectations and wanted to balance it out this way. I couldn't be that person who went ahead and did things against their approval. This has been my problem for a really long time, and even now I need them to be okay with what I do on some level.

I wanted to mention before going further to discuss my own phase of depression in this chapter that if you or anyone you know is in any kind of emotional and psychological distress, facing abuse, experiencing depression or exhibiting signs of depression, they must seek professional help from qualified and trained mental health professionals.

Here are some online counselling services that might be helpful:

https://www.snehacounselling.org/
https://icallhelpline.org/
https://www.thelivelovelaughfoundation.org/

I know I am not alone in having felt this way in the past. There are many of you living your life the same way, settling for something that you don't want to, either at work or in life, because of that fear of dealing with the people around you. Having struggled with it for a long time, I felt it's important for me to state that you are not alone in your struggles. If me opening up and talking about it in my book helps you push yourself to navigate and arrive at something in your life, I feel that's it's totally worth it to show my vulnerable side here.

Like every girl, I had my own set of dreams about marriage, a partner and to be able to live happily ever after. But when I finally did get married almost a decade back, that illusion was promptly shattered. I don't want to get into the details of my marriage here, but all I want to ask is this: Do you think anyone would get married with the intention of walking out? Who else, apart from the two people in the relationship, is affected more when and if they choose to end it?

The way I was approached about my divorce was very mournful. I agree with the idea that it is the end of a relationship and not the end of life itself. Treating divorce otherwise eliminates the opportunity for us to feel a sense of rebirth, a chance to restart life.

While I was already in a state of shock about what was happening in my marriage, what made it even worse was the backlash of harsh and crude comments that I had to endure. Until then, social media had not been a terrible experience for me. It was also the time when anyone with a social media account would freely provide their unsolicited opinions. It was a crucial, devastating phase of my life; for the first time, the ugly sides of it hit me while I was at my weakest.

At this juncture, I have to make a special mention of the YouTube channels, publications and websites that decided to have a field day with this low point in my personal life. They wrote and said all kinds of things, twisting facts around and cooking up their own stories to make me appear like a stereotypical villainess we see in films. They tarnished my public image in many ways, just to get some extra likes, views and clicks. The abuse poured in like a stream after that.

Sadly, my mom and dad, who had nothing to do with this, had to bear the repercussions too, only because their daughter was in the media industry. Up until then, they had never hung their head low for me, and even though I hadn't let them down, they felt embarrassed and hurt to handle this part of my life. They were sad for me and what I was going through, but seeing them so helpless made me feel even more miserable. We didn't know what to do and how to cope with this.

People who hardly knew me were calling me, impolitely asking if what they'd read was true and why I'd chosen to do it. Talk about crossing boundaries and stepping over the limits! People without divorces would say things like, 'Oh! I'm so sorry, but you could have waited and tried more to work things out', or 'Life is going to be very difficult after this for you', or 'Aren't you afraid about being alone forever?' On the other hand, people with divorces would congratulate me, so the entire subject was very confusing and I felt very uncomfortable throughout this period.

This phase taught me a lot of things about people. I realized that these critical opinions from people who were nosy and intrusive were nothing but projections of their own emotions, and that they were questioning me because they wanted to hear from me all that they kept pondering about their own marriage. There is another group of people who I had considered to be my close friends, but some of them just disappeared at this point in my life. They didn't return until all the drama had ended, so that they wouldn't have to be involved with me while I was going through this ordeal. The hard truth I learnt is that you are alone in the journey of life, and you must be your best friend no matter how many wonderful people, whether friends or family members, you have around you.

The effects that my short-lived marriage had on me were traumatic in every part of my life. I went into a severe state of depression. The anxiety of how to face people in public after this, the constant inner battle and self-doubt about whether I should have stayed unhappy in the marriage instead of facing all this was destroying my peace. I am a big fan of crying and mourning if one needs to express their emotions, but this was not something I could just cry and be done with. I had several meltdowns every now and then. From insomnia to constant blood pressure fluctuations, this was a phase of my life when even consecutive sessions with therapists and antidepressants were of little help. When I hit rock bottom, my thought process went through several stages:

Stage 1: Self-pity—Why me? I had everything working for me. Why did I, of all people, have to face such a situation?

Stage 2: Blame game—This happened to me not because of something I had done but because of other individuals or external circumstances.

Stage 3: I didn't deserve this—I had been a disciplined, sincere, respectful and civilized individual throughout my life. I had worked hard to get to where I was, both in my life and in my career. I had never pulled someone else down to get to the top, nor had I consciously done anything to hurt another person. Then how could things work against me? Only good things should happen to good people.

Now I realize, all these ideas and approaches that I had then were wrong.

Keeping myself busy all the time, to escape from thinking about this, was one of my initial coping mechanisms. I wanted to avoid facing the truth and address what was going on inside me and being alone felt so uncomfortable that I would always have something planned and always be on the go.

Unfortunately, the sadness just kept coming back after brief breaks, and it made me more miserable. I was feeling fatigued all the time and something told me that I wasn't handling the depression the right way. I know how many of us tend to brush it under the carpet and let ourselves become numb and live that way forever or bottle it up too long only to explode. This is exactly why talking to someone you really trust and seeking professional help is so important when it comes to the subject of depression.

The first step in fixing things and shifting my mindset was when I started to grieve for my pain. I acknowledged the fact that my marriage had ended, that it was hurtful and that it meant dismantling of a lot of connections, friendships and plans. It was an important step. I made sure I released all those bottled feelings out as much as I needed to. I offer the same advice to close friends of mine after their break ups. I simply tell them to call me when they don't feel like getting out of bed even two weeks later. I know what that feels like. The more you ignore it, the harder it comes back to bite you. I isolated myself and cried while binge watching random shows on the television. Eventually, tapping into my unhappiness and being comfortable about the sense of discomfort was very helpful.

The second step in healing was harnessing the idea that I now had a new opportunity for a fresh start. Unfortunately, women are conditioned to believe that marriage is equivalent to life itself, when in reality it's just one part of our whole life. A lot of women whose long-term marriages end feel that they don't even know who they are anymore, because they had made that marriage and relationship their whole life. I understood that I could return to living life for myself, and perhaps someone else would even come into my life at a later stage. But this was an opportunity that not everybody gets, and I realized that that was a very special thing. I remembered that while I had been married, my mother had asked me to comply with several norms to be in the good books of the ones I needed to please and be in approval of, but now I could just tie my hair up, wear my pajamas and play music in my room. This was my life now, and I could live it my way.

Thirdly, I started journalling. It helped me to not forget my experiences from my marriage, and the lessons I'd learnt from them. I wrote about the kind of person I wanted to be in the next couple of years, the changes I needed to make personally, how I could be healthier and what I could do to be happier. Writing it all down gave me a sense of clarity, and it helped me feel driven to move ahead in as positive a manner as possible.

I do believe that the universe manifests what you truly believe and want. Life has changed so much for me in all the years since then, and many of the changes I'd wanted happened in the exact manner as what I'd written down on a piece of paper when my life was crumbling around me. I have pinned that piece of paper to my dressing room mirror, and it amazes me when I look at it once in a while to realize how a lot of my wishes have come true even without my conscious efforts! I told myself that I deserved all of it, and that's all I'd contributed towards those goals. But writing down my intentions totally helped me shift my mindset in the long run.

Also, when I became comfortable with being alone, I sensed the true meaning of resilience for the first time. While society tells us that women in particular need to have a partner, I realized that it was untrue in our times, where women are as career-driven as men. Unless you have these realizations by yourself, it can be a very fearful time. I don't feel lonely nowadays when I am alone, rather it is the opposite, I crave for my me time, and that is a beautiful thing. I feel happy being on my own and watching TV, reading a book or eating a snack— loneliness is when you no longer feel the joy in being alone.

Learning from my past has helped me move forward with a lot more strength and confidence about myself. Looking back on those times today, I am proud I took charge of my life at the right time. There is nothing that feels impossible to endure anymore.

I hope that eventually the end of a marriage is as normalized as losing a job. It is hard when we lose a job that we have been a part of for many years and it lets us down emotionally, but we never grieve over it like it is the end of everything. In the same way, we just need to take the lessons from the end of a marriage and move forward, trusting in what awaits us in our future.

If there is one message I can share with those who are in a challenging marriage and are reading this chapter, it is this: Yes, your life as you knew it might have been dismantled, but remember that your marriage is only a chapter in your story, just like this a chapter in my book. It is not my entire story.

31

Social Media Toxicity

When I'd started out in media, there was no social media. The first customary ritual when you enter the entertainment industry was to get some heads shots or 'professional portfolios', as we used to call them, made spending a chunk of money on popular photographers a must. I then had to carry the portfolio around to model coordinators who would have hundreds of such portfolios already piled up on their desks. Finding the contacts of these coordinators through friends, fixing an appointment and meeting them in person (mailing won't do then), introducing myself to them and reminding them to find work for me was all I could do back then to expand and network and find my way into the modelling industry to be a part of commercials, print ads and more.

Now, social media has become a great place to showcase your talent and let people discover you. It also provides several opportunities. You cannot just introduce yourself in a generic manner, but neither do you have to trust a middleman or anyone else to make your way around the platform. You don't have to reach out to people; they can discover you and even come find you on their own if you have exactly what they want for an assignment. If I want to share something about myself, it's a lot easier now as I can do it with the click of a button, through a tweet or a post on Instagram. There is no requirement for fancy press meets, audio launches and film events to circulate news. It is rather the other way around, where we make announcements through our social media accounts. These announcements, in turn, are reported in news articles.

In spite of all these privileges, I still think that the era before this, where social media did not dominate our lives, was more peaceful.

When I introduce myself to someone today who doesn't know me, before I meet them for the second time, they get to find out about me by using Google and checking out all that the Internet has to say about me. This removes the opportunity to find out more about people organically by spending time with them.

Thus, they usually form opinions about me without giving me a chance to interact with them.

I also feel disturbed when acquaintances randomly keep probing me to follow them back or tag their social media handles from my account. Some of my 'friends' even get upset that I do not wish them publicly on Instagram, even when I make a more personal wish over a call!

Then there is the layer of professional associations as a social media influencer—I must keep putting up new content on my YouTube channel and on Instagram continuously to stay in the groove and cater to the audience which follows me. This needs to happen consistently as well because otherwise the brands that I endorse on social media would be concerned about the number of likes and engagements with my posts will decrease if I am not active and relevant on the platform.

Imagine what would happen if Instagram and Facebook removed the option to like or comment on posts, and only had the direct messaging (DM) feature? There would be a complete shift in the way the medium is approached, right? I used to keep thinking about this when I used to read disturbing comments. Everything would change—the hateful commenting would disappear, and different brands might not want to promote their products or services using the medium because the engagement rate would be a lot lower. Negativity thrives and sells like nothing else on social media.

All these social media platforms have their ways of sucking us in and then making us want more until we are caught up using the platform. I might externally say that I don't care about the number of people who like my posts, but when my make-up artist or photographer texts me and informs me that my latest post did well in terms of engagement, there is always a part of me that is curious to find out what they're talking about and check the responses to my posts. There was someone who recently contacted me by saying that they wanted to approach me for a brand deal, and the value that they were supposed to offer me for a post about the brand on my Instagram account was equivalent to the number of followers I had back then. For example, they offered me 'x' rupees for every ten followers. I refused their offer, as I didn't want to fall prey to this and get the urge to increase my follower count due to the brand deal. I am aware that there is an option to pay money and falsely increase your following as well as the likes you get on each of your posts, but thankfully I have never felt the need to pursue something like that. There is so much day-to-day work that goes on behind the scenes to run every account that I have on social media. No matter how tough and tedious it gets, I handle them on my own and do it only because of one reason. You make this so worth it. I truly appreciate it so much when you try my workouts and recipes and come back saying a thank you, share lovely things about my photoshoots, encourage and support me at my job, leave your reviews; this side of you truly makes me feel like you are part of my life and I have a very big family here on social media. So at this point, I'm taking a minute to say thank you to my one million IG, 4 lakh YouTube and 1.5 million-strong Twitter family. It's not about these numbers really, but you made the decision to become a part of this family that I have built here and have decided to stay. A MILLION people care to be with me here. That fills me with pride and happiness.

Today, success is measured by our social media posts and engagement, whether it's to do with our relationships, our body goals or lifestyles. A friend in the film industry takes her photographer to every place she travels to with her friends and family (including international locations); she shops for clothes and makes her itinerary based on what her Instagram posts will be, so that they fit a certain aesthetic on her profile. I for one used to get anxious if I didn't have any ideas or photos to post for a few days.

As long as social media activity is within the limits of what we enjoy, it is perfectly fine. These platforms can totally be a place to seek and provide inspiration and creativity, but dwelling on something and emulating others is what affects people negatively. I too have felt that in the past. Someone being happy and celebrating when I am not having a great day would ruin my day further. I would try to show myself in the best light possible, and cover up all my bad days to make it look like my life is forever rosy and beautiful, when in reality we all know that that is impossible. The real change with respect to social media happened during the pandemic last year, when I became disinterested in it, and would not engage in it as frequently as before. When I gradually cut down on my scrolling time on social media, there was a definite positive shift in my life.

My approach to social media now is that I try to post about my bad days as well. When I was extremely depressed for a long time after my pet dog Milo (you will read about him in the next chapter) passed away, I shared the news on social media. When someone shares a personal story, asking me to give them some positivity to face their situation, I don't reveal their identity but share my thoughts on it in a video post, so that it resonates with them as well as others who might be going through the same thing. When I need to take a break, I post about it on social media and do not attempt to hide my struggles. To my surprise, all of this actually gave me much more respect and adoration from my genuine followers who don't stop expressing their love over messages and emails. These days, because of these changes, I am able to connect to my audience at a much deeper level.

I personally choose to follow people who have a similar approach too, people who are themselves and do not put on an act for the sake of social media. People tend to gravitate towards and draw inspiration from those who are confident, cool and express themselves freely. It's very liberating to be in what I call a '*mafti* mindset' (*mafti* is typically when you can wear what you want and not be in the uniform you are expected to wear).

Make that change. Stop doing things that pull your spirits down. Surround yourself with good people who lift you up. Face your own truth. Believe me, the way you eat and the choices you make in your relationships and career all impact your lifestyle and health.

Use the hashtag #MaftiMindset and put up a post about something you really feel like sharing after reading this chapter, and tag me @ramyasub on Instagram. It can be anything that you didn't want to share out of your fear of being judged, but which you simply feel like expressing today.

Here's a list of things you could say and things you shouldn't say to someone when they're depressed:

DO NOT SAY THIS ✗	INSTEAD SAY THIS ✓
I know how you feel.	I'm here for you if and whenever you feel like talking about it.
It's just another bad day.	Let's go out and do something to get this off your mind.
Be positive.	It's okay if you don't feel like doing anything.
You're lucky. Think about all those people in a worse state than you.	Shall we go visit a counsellor to help ease things?
You're making a mountain out of a molehill.	I love you, no matter what.

Your Happiness Challenge

Day 1	Listen to music from your childhood. Music connects with the soul and can elevate the mood instantly. Choose happy songs please.
Day 2	Do something different today. Break your usual routine and do something you genuinely enjoy.
Day 3	Listen, read or watch something that resonates with you. It can be an old film or a book that you want to read again, to feel reassured by the good times that are soon to come in your life.
Day 4	Call a friend you trust and simply chat with them about what you're going through.
Day 5	Help someone with anything that you can. Volunteering or even donating blood counts here. The sense of satisfaction it gives is boundless.
Day 6	Have a morning regime. Watch the sun rise, meditate and show gratitude.
Day 7	Exercise to release your toxins.
Day 8	Compliment someone or simply smile at the new faces you bump into. A cheerful 'good morning' can be powerful to the other person and you.
Day 9	Do something creative and learn a new hobby. You could try your hand at a skill you lost touch with in all the hustle, or learn something online. You could even get inventive in the kitchen.
Day 10	Play your favourite song and dance like nobody's watching! Just do it.

32

My Love—Milo

This is probably a chapter that will resonate more with you if you have had a pet. While I have talked about self-care, healing, transformation and relationships, this book will be incomplete for me if I do not write about my dog Milo. For those of you who have already been following me on social media for long, Milo needs no introduction. For those of you who don't, Milo was my beloved pet, and I lost him at the beginning of the pandemic in March 2020. I got him when he was a 45-day-old puppy, early in 2011, and I remember the day he ran and jumped into my hands out of all the other puppies that were around. He became the closest one to my heart since then. I am weeping even as I write this chapter.

I have always been a dog person thanks to my dad. All of them have been German shepherds, including Milo, and this was a conscious choice because we are always reminded of the previous one we lost with the next one who comes to us. In short, all the ones we had before Milo (Tiger, Tommy and Cadbury) were mainly watchdogs, and my role was limited to bonding with them as a playmate, whereas when it was Milo's turn to come home, I had to do a lot of convincing and pleading with my parents since they wanted to cut short any added responsibilities. By that point, I realized I couldn't live in a home without a pet. I always keep thinking how unlike humans, animals don't have the luxury of expressing how they feel through words, and one needs to know it all from their eyes; so I always watch a bit more carefully when it comes to animals and their sufferings. I took it upon me to be Milo's 'dog mom' in all ways, and I always did my best.

Milo was not just my companion, and this might sound cheesy, but he was like my soulmate in every way. I learnt how to feed him, take him on walks every day, when to take him to the vet for vaccinations and check-ups, how to bathe him and how to take care of him when he was ill. We went through so much together when he was growing up. The relationship I had with Milo has been significant and therapeutic on so many levels. Being Milo's mom made me a better, responsible and more patient person. I loved him so much, and I still do. He was with me for a decade, and I still cannot imagine that he is no longer with us now. He was with me at a time when I had all these drastic changes happening in my life. During my good days, I would play a song and dance with him, get him some extra treats, and during my bad days, I would just sit next to him and he would place his paw on my lap and look at me like he knew what I was going through. Honestly, that's all I needed to feel better. There was this unsaid connection I had with Milo, which I also have now with Hero (Hero came home following Milo's demise and is two years old now). They don't need to say anything, and yet they convey what they need to with that silence. I feel like I grew up to be a more mature person with Milo. Other than the times I travelled, he was right by my side every day, from the time I woke up and took him on a walk to the time I would bid him good night and let him roam outside in the lawn before going to bed. This void in my life without him is unbearable even now.

I was a complete mess after Milo's demise. Since this happened during the intense lockdown, none of my friends could comfort me physically nor could I do anything to distract myself to heal. A few good souls did whatever they could even then, like my friend Vetri, who managed to send his puppy for me to foster to keep my mind off my own fellow.

I would have both good and bad days—sometimes, I would be happy, but I'd suddenly be reminded of Milo and have another breakdown. I missed him so much, and looking at every spot in my house would take me back to the moments we shared, how we bonded, how he would wait for me to give him treats at the kitchen corner and how he would start indicating that he wanted to play fetch with me whenever I was near the place next to the entrance where he knew I kept his toys. Milo loved car rides, and every time I sat in a car he would bark to remind me to mark a time just to take him on a drive. When I'd come home after travelling, he would jump on me and lick me all over, starting with a series of low barks that would increase in volume as he got more and more excited on seeing me (I see all these exact signs with Hero too). He was so protective of me, and whenever a stranger approached me outside our home, he would bark at them and threaten them to stay back. Milo was irreplaceable. Our love can't be described in words. I wonder what we humans do so to deserve this kind of unconditional love and such loyalty from dogs.

Though my playful little Hero can never be compared to Milo entirely, and they're both strikingly unique, I believe that Hero is blessed and was bestowed on me by Milo.

Milo did appear in my meditations soon after his life ended, and the message he gave me was to focus on the happy moments that I'd had with him instead of his sudden demise. He told me that he had chosen to do the same and that it was important for me to know that he was very grateful and blessed to have spent time with me during his life. He told me he was lucky to have a beautiful home, and that he was lucky to have me as well. He asked me to open my heart to both love and grief, and told me to allow myself to grieve for him in my own way and in my own time instead of running away from it. He told me not to feel guilty, and that I had done the best I could for him. He told me that my life would be good, with him always protecting me and being by my side, in ways different from how it used to be before.

To my sweet baby, my dear Milo, I hope that you are now resting in peace. Remember that there isn't a single day that goes by without mommy thinking about you.

33

Don't Stress While You're Stressed, or Stress to De-stress

Do you feel stressed trying to understand the title of this chapter?

If there is a survey conducted about the most commonly used word these days, it would probably be 'stress'. The word gets thrown around in every context, both by kids and adults, so much so that I sometimes wonder what it really means.

- 'Why did you not finish your homework?'
- 'I was stressed.'
- 'Why are you shopping so much?'
- 'I'm super stressed out. '
- 'Why are you not eating?'
- 'I feel stressed.'
- 'Why are you eating?'
- 'I'm stress eating!'

Whew! Now I'm stressed thinking about all the other situations that stress people out!

Basically, anything that makes us anxious, depressed, uneasy, sad, fearful or overwhelmed leads to 'stress'.

I know of certain people who, while going through bad fights with their spouses and friends or even while being bankrupt, continue to share generic 'Happy Marriage' or 'Best Friend Forever' posts, or even pictures from vacations. I guess one can't blame them when there is so much pressure to show the best version of ourselves on social media.

I agree that it's important to be happy, but I as a person cannot portray a version of myself that's completely out of sync with reality. This doesn't mean I will share my deep and personal troubles on social media, but I'm saying that it's okay to take time off social media when things aren't great or share the real reflections of what it's like to be at such a point. I try and take a deep breath, fix my problems in order of their priority and then come back to share genuine posts about my happiness.

When I sense that the day isn't going my way, I try not to get too worked up. As a general rule, I stay away from gadgets and social media on those days. It helps me stay calm and be more productive. Sometimes, just seeing another person's post and comparing our situations can provoke anxiety and make me feel insecure, so staying off social media helps. I instead spend more time on myself, focus on what is bothering me and work on fixing it. Silence is a true healer to my senses.

At a time when the pandemic is making us realize that anything can happen in a moment to us and our loved ones, and giving us a sense of constant uncertainty when dealing with our lives and careers at large, this rise of stress and other mental health issues is a serious reminder to check and fix what we need for the sake of our own health.

Most of the time, we create problems that never even existed in the first place by overthinking things, and that is just the beginning of stressing ourselves out. I, for one, am guilty of doing this. The issue is that it's not only us, but even those who love us dearly who don't know how to deal with a person when they say that they feel stressed out. The word is so generously used nowadays that we honestly don't know how to react when someone tells us that they are stressed.

When I used to tell my mom that I was stressed, she would simply ask me to relax and stop working, not realizing that my work was only contributing to the stress more but doing that would not make the stress disappear. Also, for women of that generation, their careers were not that big a deal. Not as much as looking after the family and home for sure. I used to feel upset whenever she said that to me and eventually stopped telling her for I knew she won't be able to relate to this.

On the other hand, with men I have sensed that they feel the need to be solution providers and solve things when we share what we feel (at least from my share of experiences in most cases, but of course there will be exceptions). So, when I'd tell a close male friend about my problems, he would either mostly divert my thoughts by changing the topic or try to cheer me up by providing his opinions on how to handle the situation. None of this would make me feel any better.

What we actually want sometimes is for someone to just sit with us and hear us out. Or simply let us be alone if we prefer that and not bother until we get back to normal. That's all.

Support and solidarity, politeness and positivity—this is what we need from someone who knows we are stressed. Giving that space to be able to say what someone feels when they are going through a tough situation is more valuable than doing something unsolicited.

The voices in our heads should not be telling us what to do, we should be controlling what we hear from them and process them in a more sensible and sensitive way before expressing ourselves when talking to someone who feels bothered about something. I am a clear victim of this all the time, for I often tend to overthink things because of all these voices. This tendency also arises from a part of me that wants to be a perfectionist in certain things. Especially as someone running a business of being a fitness entrepreneur for the first time ever, micromanaging every area of administration and my inherent need to execute everything perfectly—for example, the way I want my clients to have their workouts and materials for their programme sent, the way a post I share has to look in my eyes, or even the way my food is kept on the plate, zaps every bit of energy in me day in and out. I have also noticed that being this way holds me back. Instead of focusing on how to simply get things done, I would feel distracted and completely spent. My inner voice at most times hence is a pain, distraction and barrier for me and you have to hear it loud yourself (if there is a way for that) to understand the intensity of the constantly shattering noise in my head at times of stress, which even affects my sleep. Do you relate to this? What's fascinating for me is that whenever I immerse myself in spiritual teachings, I find that most gurus talk about how they channelized their inner voices effectively into becoming who they are. I also realized during the lockdown that when I was doing something that I enjoyed or having fun with people, my inner voice was silent, because I was too focused at the task at hand. But while I was at home with all the restrictions, not being able to go out anywhere or do anything, the isolation made my inner voice act up far too often. I was crumbling from within on just hearing it.

If we listen to ourselves, be mindful of what we are thinking and slow down a bit, that's when we tend to realize what the real problem is.

Whenever I find myself in a stressful situation these days, I try and approach it in different ways on my own by doing the following:

- I talk to myself about the situation, alone in a room, and try to figure out a way to handle it mentally so that it's resolved and I can move on (make sure you are alone in the room when you do this—if someone sees you talking to yourself, they'll think you've completely lost it due to all that stress!). This helps 90 per cent of the time.

- I divert my mind by doing something completely unrelated taking tiny little breaks that gives me a new burst of energy when I get back to work again.

- I turn off my mobile data or sometimes put my phone on Airplane mode as it affects the quality and efficiency of my work.

- When the anxiety melts away and I feel sane again, I take a few deep breaths and ask myself what I can change to avoid this from happening the next time. Then, I take proactive steps to avoid a repetition of the same scenario.

Apart from smaller bouts of stress, I've also faced major panic attacks in the past when I started anchoring events other than TV shows (which were confined to limited crew and most of the talk was to the camera), especially when I've had to host shows in front of large gatherings. There was a time when I'd feel extremely flustered and scared exactly a few minutes before going onstage. Getting a hundred instructions from all corners and having changes made to my script at the very last moment would make things worse. Even little things, like the mic not working properly, would bother me a lot. If things that were beyond my control went wrong, I would take it personally. The lights going off, a sudden downpour just before an outdoor show, sleazy comments from the audience, cringy remarks made on my clothes and appearance by a co-host, screeching mics, an LED screen failure or a mix-up of participants onstage—all of these would irk me to no end.

Fear can affect us in different ways. It can motivate us to do courageous acts—for instance, it helps me prepare well for a powerlifting competition, or when I audition for a role in a film, when I have scenes with a senior actor in a film and I don't want to make mistakes, etc. Recently, I tied up with Film Companion, one of India's leading Entertainment YouTube Platforms, for a few months as their South face for conversations with film personalities. The excitement-mixed adrenaline rush for me was to go back to being an interviewer; researching and watching films related to the celebrities I connected with; getting the finer details right to make my conversations with celebrities more engaging for *The Ramya Show*—all of it scared me in a good way.

Fear is also capable of paralysing me—in the past, I have frozen in fear just before a dance performance, even after all the innumerable hours of rehearsing the steps. At various points in time, I have also realized that one of the demands of my job is to buckle up and endure my fear. I could be an exceptional actor, but if I can't pull myself together and give an audition where all the eyes in a room are on me, that'd be the end of my career.

One day, I took some time to reflect on my stress. It wasn't doing my health nor my work any good, and it certainly wasn't bringing out the best in me. It was affecting the way I worked with my team, and the stress would also show on camera. I didn't like the way I appeared, nor was I having fun doing the job that I loved so much. I don't have a job where I have the choice to work in isolation. Being an anchor or an actor, and now a health coach, is all about getting comfortable with the crowd and building resilience to face the camera or look at thousands of people in the eye and talk, emote, dance or exercise.

So, what could I do to manage this? I decided to calm myself down and set aside a few minutes before every event, just to focus on myself and my peace of mind. This meant I would start getting my make-up done a little earlier. When I was fully ready, I would inform my team that I'd be back in just a few minutes, asking them to not look for me or be worried, and then go lock myself up somewhere. I'd close my eyes, say a little prayer, think of a few happy memories, listen to some good music, practise my power poses in front of the mirror, and take nice, long, deep breaths. And when I knew I was completely calm and collected, I opened my eyes, wished

myself the very best, and then went ba
chaos, giving all my energy to the peop
me. Most importantly, I enjoyed the m
to the absolute fullest. After all, I'm gra
opportunities and would like to fully en
one day I can look back at it all and think fondly about all I've
done.

The margin of error in something that is stressful for us
totally depends on how we think of it in our heads. It manifests
positively or negatively based on how I decide, and that's how
I choose to understand this. The first step is to realize that all
these doubts, anxieties and worries that I face is not the actual
reality, but mere thoughts.

Even if this was not about work but simply about not
wanting to wake up in the morning early, get out of the
bed and go do a workout at home during times of stress and
uncertainty during the lockdown, as much as it was hard for
me to get started on it, this was the only thought that reassured
me and helped me then to trick my mind and snap out of any
negative thoughts.

I also realized why exercise, or an outdoor hike, or
photography or any other hobby that we enjoy actually makes
us feel excited—because it makes our bodies and mind rest
while we focus in the moment. Exercise distracts our mind with
all the physical labour that we are involved in while working
out. The mind is so busy working in the moment of enduring
the physical hurdle that it can't distract you in any other way.
Even meditation works according to the same principle of not
cancelling or shutting our thoughts out, but noticing the mind
wandering and bringing it back to focus. Just a few minutes of

...ce and meditation have had remarkable effects on me over ...me. I feel more positive, refreshed and able to productively manage the day-to-day tasks. I feel more excited to do my job, and I don't remember the last time when I was not in control of my feelings since I started meditating religiously. It has removed my fatigue, and I no longer feel dazed. It gives a sense of balance to look at ourselves from outside our body. This is why it is therapeutic to do things we love.

Here's a list of things I constantly do to live in the moment and shut out all the noise:

- I try to play badminton at least once a week. Every time I play, my mood elevates to levels of bliss. A good morning starts with great company and makes for a happy day.
- Going for an early morning or late evening jog amidst nature in a park or beach, while listening to some good music or podcast. I simply forget everything else.
- Experimenting and innovating in the kitchen with recipes.
- Sometimes, when I need a break from my routine, I try taking a day off and going somewhere on my own. Being in a new place by myself, eating the local street food, talking to strangers I meet while travelling—all of it helps me reflect and appreciate what I have in my life.

Have any of you guys ever seen me watching movies by myself at Sathyam Cinemas? As much as I enjoy watching films with a group of friends, I often take off on my own to watch films too—We are our worst enemy, and it's totally up to us to either make the monster an angel or let it continue to disrupt our lives. The next time you get stressed, just allow yourself to breathe and say that it's okay to feel that way for starters. The rest shall follow in time.

Exercise

Write about an unforgettably stressful situation in your life. How did you deal with it, and how do you think you would deal with it more effectively the next time?

_____

_____

_____

_____

_____

34

Mirror, Mirror on the Wall

Being in a profession that demands you look good all the time can take a toll on you. It's no easy task to wake up to this kind of pressure every single day of your life, and to endure it every time you step out of the house (or even while you're at home, thanks to social media!). The occupational hazard of being in the public eye is that how we look, what we wear and what we do is under constant scrutiny.

When I was 15 years old and in the early stages of my career, all of this took a toll on me. I remember the days when people pointed fingers at me when I walked by and made snide remarks. Some of them even had offensive nicknames for me. The constant criticism was extremely difficult to deal with. But years of being exposed to this sort of harassment helps you develop a tough exterior and take things in a lighter vein.

The simple routine that I follow now is to look at myself in the mirror every morning and say, 'I love you'. I tell myself that despite the challenges the day might bring, I will not lose my cool; I'll stay calm and keep smiling. I will treat myself better and be kinder, not just to others, but to myself too.

Criticizing someone is the easiest thing to do; however, getting over harsh and unwarranted criticism from somebody else is the hardest thing to do, even if their remark might contain a grain of truth. While I agree that you should be able to take yourself lightly and laugh things off, certain boundaries need to be clearly defined in every relationship. Nobody should be allowed to take a jab at you or how you look, no matter who you are or how close that person is to you.

For a long time after I started my career in front of the camera, I was told by random people that I need to lose weight. When I started exercising, I was told that I do 'too much cardio', which isn't good for my physique, and that I had to stop lifting weights when I was into powerlifting, in case I became too muscular and started to look too manly. The latest piece of advice was that I've become too lean and need to add some weight 'in the right places' to look more appealing. Sigh!

Honestly, I wouldn't change a thing about any of these 'looks' I've had at various points in my life. Each one of them has shaped my confidence and has progressively taught me to love my body. They've also given me the most important lesson of my life, which is: Don't let anyone define how you should look!

I'm sure that many of you have your own stories of hurtful remarks that have affected your body image in some way. Some time ago, my make-up artist confided in me about her struggle to lose her post-pregnancy weight. She'd run into a friend at a wedding and the first thing he said was '*Ennadi, panni maaduriaayitta*!' ('You look like a pig!') She was hurt and embarrassed, but swallowed her feelings and simply responded with a smile. My heart went out to her—she had tears in her eyes when she shared this with me.

If you, dear reader, have ever been hurt by someone else's inconsiderate words, I send you my tightest hug, firstly. Secondly, no matter who this person is, you need to rethink their place in your life. Also, please bear in mind that you can never stop others' comments, for that is one thing that is not in your control. All you can do is become mentally stronger as a person. While most of us think that this confidence can only come once we reach our goals, I can assure you that it never made any difference to me when I reached my goals. The confidence and happiness you lack is nothing to do with the way you look. The process you undertake to get healthy can be a stimulant in pushing your boundaries and knowing your capacities—I agree with that, but you should work on being confident now with how things are at present, rather than be trapped in the web of comments made about you. This is how I overcame the body shaming that happened and still happens to me. It isn't easy, and it can't happen overnight. However, have faith in yourself and trust the process, for I did eventually overcome it. If I could do it, so can you!

Finally, if you happen to be that person who casually makes fun of your friends or partner for how they look, here's a word of caution: you might think that this is a fun way to get closer to them and have a few laughs, but your 'harmless' comments could have long-term damaging effects on their self-image and self-worth and will slowly destroy your relationship.

There's a saying that goes, 'No matter how dark the night, morning always comes, and our journey begins anew.' Tomorrow onwards, I want you to wake up with a smile on your face. Put your mobile phones aside, walk straight to the mirror, look yourself in the eye and talk to yourself in a positive, reaffirming way. Remind yourself of how far you've come in your life, how beautiful you look and how blessed you have been. Feel energized before you step out of your room, and go conquer the day ahead of you!

Things I Do When I Wake Up

- I make my bed as soon as I wake up, thus accomplishing my first task of the day.
- I look at myself in the mirror, smile and give myself a pep talk.
- While having my morning drink, I visualize the kind of day I want to have, and think about my routine and meetings scheduled for the day.
- I meditate for 10 minutes. During this time, I check to see if anything is bothering me, find a way to accept it and let it go.
- I head to the gym for a quick workout, go on a walk with Hero or simply stretch for about 10–15 minutes while listening to my favourite music to help charge me up.

Exercise

Write down three things that you will say to yourself in front
of the mirror before you step out and face the world today:

1. _____
2. _____
3. _____

35

What Is Your Life's Purpose?

Why has this life been given to us? In other words, what is our life's purpose?

Finding your life's purpose is no easy task. It has to be ambitious enough to get you out of bed every morning, but it should also be realistic and completely achievable. In other words, our life's purpose needs to excite us and be within the limits of our capabilities at the same time.

As I've said, I started my career as a television anchor. I started by hosting small shows on Jaya TV when I was in the 9th grade and continued part-time hosting on and off until the 12th grade.

When I was in college, I participated in the 'Miss Chennai' beauty pageant and was one of the finalists. I was also the winner of two titles, 'Talent of Chennai' and 'Voice of Chennai'. This opened up the modelling world for me, which subsequently led to my entry into Star Vijay.

When you're in the limelight, a constant sense of doubt and insecurity hangs over you. Despite that, I was a happy teenager. The simple fact that I was working at an age when most of my classmates and seniors were only studying was a big motivator. I still remember my first salary—Rs 600—which I used to buy my mom a sari. How much I earned didn't matter so much; the feeling of accomplishment that it gave me was worth so much more.

Several years went by this way. I was happy with what I was doing and had settled into a comfort zone of sorts, with no real goal or intention to get better. I continued to take up whatever was offered to me and enjoyed the fruits of my labour.

However, about five years ago, I suddenly received a wake-up call. This happened in the period when I was hosting a show with a co-anchor. My co-anchor had gotten the opportunity to act in a film, and during a particular event we were hosting together, he made a casual remark about how so many previous anchors whom I had co-hosted the show with had become leading heroes, and that he'd soon become one too. He added that someday in the future, he would watch me co-host with the next generation of male anchors, who would also go the same route.

I'm sure he had no intention of being patronizing, but somewhere, his words implied that there had been—and would continue to be—no growth in my career beyond being a television anchor. The incident shook me up really badly. I realized that I had become so sedate with my job I'd barely even realized that it no longer excited me. It had become part of a mundane routine, almost like brushing my teeth or bathing in the morning. I had stopped pursuing anything beyond the 'safe zone'. I had a lump in my throat just thinking about it.

Though I've avoided mentioning the name of this particular co-host, I would like to thank him for what he did.

If not for that incident, I might still have been on a hamster wheel, hosting a TV show with no focus or goal ahead of me.

I understand that not everyone enjoys what they do for work, and that many people are compelled to work purely for financial stability. But no matter what you do, it is important to continually check on yourself to know how you are feeling, and to set progressive goals. Life happens so quickly; just pausing every once in a while and looking at it through a different window can help put things in perspective.

In my case, I loved hosting when I'd started, but over time, it became monotonous and stale. I needed a catalyst to shake me out of it. Eventually, I came to realize that my true fulfilment lay in showing people how remarkable life can be when you take a positive approach and break away from routine and make bold changes. It's important that your own life is filled to the brim with joy and excitement, so that you can enable people around you to enjoy the same thing.

It's something I strive to do every day.

Exercise

Have you ever thought about your life's purpose? What is the legacy that you want to leave behind? Give this some deep thought and write about it below:

_____

_____

_____

_____

_____

36

My Path Is a Distinct Path
(*EnVazhi Thani Vazhi*)

I have a habit of writing things down when they clutter up my head. It frees up my mind, so I pen down everything that occupies space there: my moods, a particular incident or encounter with someone that is bothering me, a pending task, reminders for errands and schedules for the next day. I even used to maintain a diary once upon a time, but I stopped writing and stashed it away after realizing the serious repercussions it may lead to!

There are times when I come across a list of goals that I'd written down at a certain point in the past, either a few months or years earlier. I realize how I'd subconsciously pursued a few of them, while the rest materialized in a different and much better way than how I'd originally planned! Stumbling upon these lists has been extremely rewarding at times when I'd least expected it.

My writing habit has done me a great amount of good and has extended to a 'vision board' that I've hung up in my TV room. This vision board is like an open canvas where I pin up all my dreams, ideas and goals, both short- and long-term. I even cut out inspiring articles that I read and tack them up on this board. Similarly, I have written single-line 'thoughts to myself' on sticky notes that make my room colourful. I have stuck them above my TV, on the front door, near the mirror and next to my bed—basically all the spots that my eyes can't miss. These thoughts help me get over my flaws so that I can better myself each day, bringing me a few steps closer to my goals.

Some people like to shout out their end goal and say, 'I am going to do this!' and then go out and achieve it. Putting it out there and announcing to the world that they're going to go after a particular goal helps keep them motivated.

I belong to the other category of people who prefer to work in silence and allow the end result of my work to make the noise. This is why I make no mention of my future plans. Somewhere in the back of my mind, I start to fear that I'll jinx myself when I'm overconfident about something. Having been in the media industry for so long now, I have learnt that nothing is really yours until the final product is delivered (and sometimes, things can change even after that). So, until and unless I accomplish something and fully see it through, I don't like to claim it as mine. This is also why even writing this book had been 'under the cover' for long until I decided to announce it to the world about it. I suppose everyone has their own way of doing things.

We often hear people calling themselves either a 'morning person' or a 'night person'. I've been a morning person ever since my schooldays. I'll tell you how it all began.

Call it a sign of short-term memory loss or an effect of anxiety, but I have a tendency to forget people's names, dates and other such details. Sometimes, I'll even forget people's faces and find myself unable to recollect when and where I'd seen them earlier. I guess this is inevitable due to my forever preoccupied and zoned-out state of mind which we have already addressed in the chapter about stress.

When I was in school, I was excellent at rote learning and reproducing the texts I'd learnt, but there was a catch—I had to write down everything that I'd memorized within a few hours. Otherwise, I would find it hard to retain it all in my memory.

So, I came up with a unique solution. While most of my friends would study till midnight on the eve of the exam, get some rest, wake up and get ready the next morning then head to the examination hall, I would sleep by 8:30 or 9 p.m. on the previous night and then wake up at around 2 a.m. in the morning. I'd keep studying till the very last moment, just so I could immediately pour out everything that I'd learnt! That was also when I figured that I tend to perform well under pressure.

I know that for most of you reading this now, my unique way of approaching exams isn't relatable. But that's okay. It's through things like these that we realize how distinctly different we all are from one another. If I had felt weird about setting up a system for myself this way and simply followed what all my other classmates were doing, I probably might not have scored as much as I did—not because I had a memory problem, but because I wouldn't have felt the confidence in adapting to a routine that wasn't for me.

Life is constantly going to prompt us to fit in, and it's important that we say no sometimes, when the voice inside us senses that what everyone else is doing won't quite work for us. My parents would have probably been happier if I did a basic degree, got married and was 'settled' at this stage of my life. But

I did something right by listening to my gut and choosing to live out my choices and decisions. And it did work out pretty well for me, right? By God's grace and the blessings of people who rooted for me, I have done well for myself both in my career and personally as a human being than what I would have been able to do if I had simply gone down the same path as the rest.

Most of us prefer to tag along with the crowd, just because it's easier to do that. But our distinct, individual lives have been given to us to allow each one of us to make a difference; to make individual choices, chase our own goals, live our own dreams and do things our own way. It isn't easy for sure, but you get stronger and more confident as you go along. Never try to blend in and always be proud of the unique person that you were created to be.

Exercise

List down your top three long-term goals (to be accomplished five years from now):

1. _____
2. _____
3. _____

List down your top three short-term goals (to be accomplished in the next six months):

1. _____
2. _____
3. _____

37

Be Your Biggest Fan

Being consistent while working towards something you want to achieve gets harder when there's a lack of motivation and appreciation. But it's precisely during such times that you need to clap for yourself to keep going. This is a lesson I've learnt from my mom.

Our moms are unicorns who hustle day in and day out, expecting nothing in return for all that they do and sacrifice. My mom is truly one such rock star. She started cooking for her entire family when she was only 9 years old.

However, at home we feel so entitled about this that we hardly make a mention of her excellent cooking skills. Even when we particularly relish something that she has prepared, we don't tell her that we loved the dish or thank her for it. We just eat and leave the table. I know I am not the only one who does this. In the patriarchal society that we live in, we take the women of the house for granted. It is expected of them to run the home and do everything to attend to everyone, but do we recognize what they do with small acts of kindness like a hug or a thank you or at least by saying that we are grateful? I don't think so. I have seen it happening in all the Indian homes I have visited so far. This is an unfortunate truth.

I used to feel terribly guilty about it, but would think getting her a nice gift whenever I can like on her birthday and Mother's Day would be good enough to compensate. That's what some of us do. But no, it simply isn't enough. Mother's Day should not become the one day of the year when mothers are seen as gods on social media—we should celebrate them as much as possible on all days of the year. And getting materialistic gifts is never going to match up to our love in the form of simple things that we do to show that we care for them—a smile, a hug, words of appreciation, warmth and kindness in our words and actions. Not once has my mom asked us at home why we don't appreciate her, nor has she taken a break from cooking because of the lack of validation from the family. She wakes up early and no matter how busy she is, she cooks with the two ingredients that not even the best chefs in the world can give us—love and care. She will call me every few hours when I am out or at work asking just the one question 'If I have had my meal'. She is the only one who will dutifully check on my brother and me asking us when we will get back home. My mom is the backbone of my family, keeping my dad, brother and me together; she is like the roots of a banyan tree. She is the binding force for us.

I owe my entire career to my mom too. I was very young when I started out, and my dad laid out a strict condition: either my mom accompanies me wherever I go or I don't do it at all. So, until a few years ago, my mom would get up early in the morning to finish all her chores, and then she would accompany me to my filming locations and sit there all throughout just to be my companion and guardian. She'd return home with me exhausted after the long day, but still find the energy to make some food, clean up, sort things out for the day and sleep for just a few hours before carrying on with the same routine the next day. If my mom hadn't supported me back then, I don't know where I would be in my life right now. I certainly wouldn't have been able to pursue a career I'm so passionate about.

For the last two years, I have been seeing a side of my mom that I had never known about. She has always been the homemaker, taking care of my father, brother and me and helping us all grow to what we have become today. While I thought that was all she wanted, the pandemic threw all of us into different situations and made me realize what my mom really wanted. As my father was a lawyer, he had to limit himself to handling his legal cases online, and I started focusing on my health coaching business and learning the art of running the home, asking my mom to take a back seat. She was so relieved on seeing me take up her role, and what she did in her newfound spare time surprised me. She asked me to help her create accounts on Zoom and Skype, and started learning to chant slogans from the Bhagavad Gita and 'Vishnu Sahasramam' and more with her group of friends virtually. Next, I signed her up for yoga sessions with a tutor. Soon, she started practising yoga on her own every day. While I thought my mom would make use of the free time to relax, I was stunned by how she used her time in the most productive way. It made me feel bad, because none of us at home ever encouraged her or have even thought of asking her if she wanted to do something for her own self in the past. Maybe my mom wanted a certain job. I remember the time when she took part in a cooking show along with me and won the first prize. She was simply overjoyed at winning a modular kitchen all on her own using her culinary skills and I could see in her eyes the sense of achievement and accomplishment. She was craving for it so badly all along. To be noticed and recognized by us, who are her world!

My mom belonged to the generation where women didn't have a say in achieving anything outside their duties at home, and it was a given that every woman's only job was to cook and clean. I actually spoke to her very recently about this and asked if she felt restricted by us in leading the life she dreamt of. All she told me was that she didn't know if there was any other path for her. She also said that everything she did was for my father, brother and me, and all of it was out of love. She did not see it as a job, so she didn't exactly feel deprived of anything.

I have also realized many times that for a very very long time my mom would not eat until my father finished his meals. She always waited to serve him his food, no matter how late it got, for long until she started having health issues and the doctor advised her to strictly take her meals on time. Despite my father telling her not to do so, she would continue the ritual she believed in even if that wasn't expected of her. I guess this was also because of her conditioning to be part of the system that existed then. Seeing her mother doing the same, my mom would have felt that this is the only way to act. Having said that, I am very happy that my mom is finally owning her life and doing what she wants to do. Now that

I can back her up, she plans short trips with her siblings and pilgrimages with her friends. I too take her out as much as I can to her kind of mini pilgrimages and bigger vacations, films, etc. to keep her happy.

It's high time we start contributing more to our mothers and fathers, without whom we wouldn't exist. It need not be a formal 'thank you' each time, but even holding them when they need to feel reassured about our intimacy with them, taking over the kitchen duties once in a while, offering to wash and clean the vessels or help them cut the vegetables and gently massaging their neck when they look stressed are a few good ideas that we can all try out. Noticing the number of old people who felt stranded during the pandemic as their kids were out of India, leaving them alone to battle sickness and old age, or even the number of elderly people living in old-age homes unattended while their kids are alive and doing well, was heartbreaking.

Since childhood, I have constantly been validated for all the skills I possessed and the way I explored them. Whether it was while taking my Bharatnatyam lessons as a child or anchoring a show on television that was watched by millions of people who sent me feedback, I was so used to that external validation that I felt upset if I didn't get appreciated for something I did.

But from observing my mother's life, what I learnt was that I am not competing with anyone but myself, and the focus should always be on how much I love what I do. It doesn't matter if I reach the end goal; I should give my best during the journey and love it every bit along the way.

Just like moms never treat their labour as a transaction and calculate how much they've done for us or what they've gained from it, if you truly love your job, you will enjoy the process rather than expect results.

Also, being your own fan is very important. I have realized from all the hard times in my life that no one is going to open the door for you if it's closed. You have to knock on it, unlock it, break it or enter through the back door—it's all about what you decide to do.

Just like my heroic mother, be a fan of yourself first and foremost, and the world will follow suit!

Exercise

List five things that you like about yourself below:

1. _____

2. _____

3. _____

4. _____

5. _____

38

Gyan and Gossip Don't Matter

Everybody has an opinion about everything we do. They judge our actions, our choices and sometimes even offer unsolicited advice. You're nodding your head in agreement right now, aren't you?

Speaking of nodding, give those neck muscles a break and do a few exercises before you continue reading. Our everyday mobility and flexibility go a long way in keeping us not just pain free, but also in increasing the range of motion in every muscle that would otherwise tighten when not in use due to age and lack of physical activity.

1. So even on days when I don't have time for any workout regime or a walk, I ensure that I don't fail to take 5 minutes at least 3–4 times a day to flex and stretch the muscles in the body. For all the constant neck bending that we do while using our mobile phones and laptops, this is a mandatory regime for each one of us to avoid spasms and stiffness: Lie down flat on the edge of the bed.

Roll a towel and place it at the base of your neck. Now, let your head fall back towards the floor. Relax and stay in this position for a couple of minutes.

2. Sit comfortably in a chair. Hold your hands behind your neck and pull your head down, bringing your chin towards your chest and tuck it in. Hold for a couple of minutes.

3. Sit on a chair. Place your right hand on top of your head and gently pull it down towards your right side. Hold for a couple of minutes. Repeat this on the opposite side.

4. Perform a doorway stretch—this helps to activate the otherwise drooping pecs and shoulders. Place both your hands on either sides of the door's entrance at right angles, and slightly lean forward to feel the stretch on your chest and shoulders.

Doesn't that feel better?

Good. Now, where were we? Judging people, yes.

I used to have publicists in the industry call me from time to time, asking if there was any 'news' I wanted to share. I used to think that they were asking about new projects or wanted titbits about an ongoing assignment, but only recently did I understand that they subtly wanted to check if I wanted to fabricate news about myself to catch some attention. So just so you know, the next time you read a news snippet about an actor being paired with a certain other co-actor or an actor being a part of a film project—remember it could be just for the news to spread and grab some attention, while putting the actor concerned in the limelight! From photographs taken at the airport to the ones outside a gym, if you think of it, everything is pre-planned 99 per cent of the time. I used to wonder how the press photographers knew well in advance that a certain actor is going to head to the airport or go to work out and wait there to take pictures of them at that specific time; but now I understand that the artist's PR team actually informs the photographers about their client's location. Even though I have been an interviewer/ moderator myself, I personally don't enjoy giving interviews and it comes as a shock whenever I have expressed it. Being a part of a channel myself, I do understand that running a media channel (YouTube/Television) is very challenging and competitive. When it comes to doing an interview, there are many factors: for example, how soon you are in the rat race of getting the celebrity's interview before any other channel. Most of time, everything is about how cringey the content can get and, of course, in a YouTube channel especially all that matters in the end is the number of views and likes generated by the video. But all the times that I did oblige and give YouTube interviews, I had bad experiences as they would use sleazy pictures for the thumbnails and provocative titles for the videos. The teasers for these interviews would make it sound like I had spoken negatively about another famous actor, making it seem like I am an unfairly critical person, just to make the video look enticing, controversial and make the audience want to watch it.

Next, I've had 'friends' whose sole purpose of meeting me would be to find out if what they'd read about a certain celebrity in a gossip column was true, and to get other juicy details on the latest gossip about the film industry or a recent celebrity couple break-up. I used to be as excited as they are when I was on the other side, but after I became recognizable and was spotted and written about a lot of times, and after putting myself into the shoes of those whom I was curious to know about, it's now too disturbing for me to consider gossiping as something harmless.

Thus, I have become a silent spectator during these gossip sessions, or I change the topic to something more positive about that person. Even if I catch myself saying something negative about someone, the minute I become aware of my words, I stop. I beg to differ in the perspective that writing or talking about a person's personal life is harmless entertainment as long as it isn't directly hurting that person. I still don't think that it is fine to do that, because I think that we show our real selves when nobody is watching us. If I am soft and kind to someone in front of them, but talk terribly about them to my friends behind their back, that is not just a character assassination, but also speaks more about my own character and how untrustworthy I am. Especially if this is a friend and celebrity. Let's say this friend let me down regarding something. I would prefer confronting them face to face about it if their actions bothered me, even at the cost of us parting ways after that, rather than talk about what they shared with me based on trust with somebody else for a moment of joy (I don't see the joy anymore either).

You might argue that this is true only if you know the person. But what if you talk about a celebrity who won't know you, nor would you ever know them personally? Doesn't the truth in what you say about the subject or person become questionable then?

I am pointing this out not because I am a saint who has never gossiped. In fact, I used to think that gossip and small talk were great ways to network and become closer to someone. But over time, and by having the right kind of people around me who added some sense into my thinking and approach towards the subject, I just don't feel good wasting precious time talking about people like that. A healthy mind does not seek pleasure through the path of emotional bullying and negativity.

Now, why am I sharing thoughts on the subject of gossip with you? This is because on the road to changing your life and lifestyle patterns, you will most definitely face stumbling blocks in the form of people who will talk about you behind your back. They might think that their words will never reach your ears, but it's a small world after all, isn't it?

It's also impossible for everyone to like us, and it's important to come to terms with the fact that there will be people who dislike us, which is perfectly fine.

This used to be hard for me to come to terms with, as I used to desperately try hard to be accepted and liked by everyone around me. That's the way we are raised at home. Be a good child, listen to everyone and obey, follow the rules, be someone who is liked by everyone. Maybe that was also why even a small and silly news on a page 3 column written about me like me being a 'repeat offender' (that I was wearing the same set of footwear at two different events within a few weeks gap) would make me flip out in the early days. I would be so devastated and cry in embarrassment about it. I'd go over those pages repeatedly, and question why I had been targeted, thinking about the number of people who would have read it and laughed thinking of me. This happened again and again until I realized that there was no end to this, and that it just wasn't worth it. I picked myself up, understanding that it is an unfair world that we live in, and that I needed to toughen up. Like I said earlier, the people around me now are those who help me dwell only in positivity. My friends helped me too in learning to form my thoughts about people by coming to know them in person, and not by what I read about them on the Internet or by face value. I am grateful and blessed for my friends that way. They have my back and I have theirs. So these days, whether it is a piece of gossip published in a newspaper or magazine, titles of a YouTube video made specifically to spread something unflattering about me or a nasty meme made by trolls, I simply keep away and stay oblivious to it all. Even if someone does bring it to my notice, I don't react much. I use it as a lesson to understand more about the person who said it and swiftly cut them out of my life.

It's a hard world out there, and to not just be a survivor but also to be in control of your life, it's a good idea to ignore certain people and things that come your way. What might seem like the end of your life now will be something you look back on years later and simply laugh about. So, it doesn't matter who thinks what about you. Just keep going like you don't care and really, don't care!

Five Techniques That Help Me
Stay Away from Gossip

1. Self-check: Understand what kind of person I want to grow into and form a set of core values.
2. Stand my ground: Stick to my core values no matter what, rather than compromise to please someone or to try and fit in.
3. Be honest: Ask myself why I want to talk about this person and address my vulnerabilities.
4. Be private: Know the difference between being rude and being private. I choose to be courteous with everyone, but I tend to be careful about sharing sensitive information that could be used against me.
5. Multiply my positive energy: Save my time and energy for those who deserve it and make myself less available to toxic people.

Exercise

All of us have gossiped and have been gossiped about. In the space below, write about the time you'd been gossiped about. How did that make you feel and what were the emotions you experienced?

_____

_____

_____

_____

_____

_____

Now, close your eyes and recollect a time when you laughed about someone behind their back, wrote a rude comment or mocked someone. Try to empathize with the person you did this to, apologize to them in your mind and let it go.

39

Don't Fall Prey to This

How many times have you sworn to yourself that you're going to stay away from all your social media platforms for a day (Twitter, Facebook, Instagram, Snapchat, ShareChat, Hello, etc.), and then end up breaking the rule within a few hours?

What is the first thing you reach for the second you open your eyes in the morning or sometimes even when you wake up in the middle of the night? What is the last thing you look at before you go to sleep? 99.9 per cent of our answers will be the same: our third hand, i.e., mobile phones. They contain everything, from personal photos, memos, bank passwords, reminders and appointments to our sleep data, water consumption data, data on bowel movements, and periods and ovulation tracking data! Parting with our mobile phones for a brief while would work most of us up into a frenzy of rage or anxiety.

I remember the days when my dad used to have this heavy, brick-shaped phone. The local charges for an outgoing call were around Rs 10 per minute back then. Technology has become much more affordable these days, with an incredible variety of offers to choose from (the flip side of this is that there is no limit to the amount of time we spend talking and texting on the phone, or surfing the Internet). In fact, many relationships seem to be hanging by a thread and surviving only thanks to mobile phones! Just think back to the peak of the COVID-19 lockdown. Would we have been able to function, survive and remain in our senses if there were no mobile phones? God is great!

When I first made accounts on Facebook, Twitter and Instagram, I did not realize nor expect even a little bit that they would later become a revenue generating model. Today there exist several creative, interesting and financially rewarding job profiles one can take up just on social media. A few that I know of are content manager, social media executive, social media analyst, public relations manager, digital brand marketing strategist, brand influencer, YouTuber and this list keeps growing. I'd like to put on record that while the revenues are great, to work with brands that I personally believe in/use in my everyday life and to connect with their vision is one of my goals. It helps me build long-term relationships and also makes me talk confidently about it with my audience.

Having said that, none of the names/brands/products/ services that I have mentioned in the book is a part of paid endorsements and any such association is only a reference of what I use personally.

The point here is, in order to keep things rolling, I have to keep my digital content engaging, so I am bound to use social media on a regular basis. These days, anyone facing the camera has to maintain a connection and visibility with their audience, to be able to grow and promote their work. In fact, many producers prefer to work with artists who have a large reach on social media, because that gives them an edge over artists who won't be able to promote their projects online.

As a result, I also end up falling into the trap of excessively using the digital space. I tell myself that 'it's all part of my work', but more often than not, it simply becomes an excuse to waste time with mindless scrolling, catching up with everyone else's new posts, tweets and stories!

However, I have recently started to become conscious of how much time I spend on my phone, and have taken steps to regulate it. I have changed the settings on my phone so that if I use them beyond the set duration, all apps get locked. If I open a particular app after that, it reminds me that I've reached my limit for the day and asks if I'd still like to continue. This prompts me to stop for a moment, think about the precious time I am wasting, and swiftly close the app.

I also keep a check on my daily screen time and have gotten into the habit of turning off my mobile data most of the time. This way, I check my WhatsApp messages only when I'm at home or in a place where I can connect to Wi-Fi. A few months back, my cousin mentioned how he feels so positive in the morning and goes to sleep at night at peace and has a no disturbance sleep after this ritual he started: it was to turn off his instant messenger apps at 8 p.m. and only turn them on at 8 a.m. I started doing the same as I was very curious to see if it made any difference to me. I have to admit, it feels good, peaceful, positive and enriching to stay gadget-free. It helps you prepare for the day ahead as well as go to sleep at the end of the day with a freer, calmer and clearer mind.

Since then, I have been following a regime of taking one day in the week, preferably Sunday, to switch off my phone completely and stay away from all external demands and distractions. I tell you, it feels so rejuvenating every time I do this. It is like a refresh button to set me up for the challenging week ahead! Even when I have a bad day or I am upset with someone or something, I prefer to quickly turn the phone to Airplane mode, take a deep breath, put the phone away and divert myself by doing something else and handle the situation a little later in a calmer way rather than act without thinking and regretting later. It helps.

A day productively spent is a day that adds to your life's entire success; a day wasted is something that has been forever taken away from your one and only lifetime. Plant this thought firmly in your mind.

Earn Your Screen Time

Try this out next Sunday: Use your gadgets only after completing the items on this checklist, for every part of the day. That's the rule. Do this for a few weeks and see for yourself how it feels:

Morning Checklist

- Brush your teeth. ☐
- Make your bed. ☐
- Do your physical activity for the day. ☐
- Finish your breakfast. ☐

Afternoon Checklist

- Complete one household chore. ☐
- Take a shower. ☐
- Read a book for at least 30 minutes. ☐
- Help prepare lunch at home. ☐
- Finish lunch. ☐

Evening Checklist

- Play with kids, walk the dog, or do some kind of physical activity for at least 30 minutes. ☐
- Write something in your journal about the week that went by. ☐
- Plan for the week ahead. List down the tasks to be accomplished at work and at home. ☐

It goes without saying that you can't check your phones an hour before you go to sleep and for an hour after waking up. Happy digital break-up!

40

It's Hard to Be a Proton in a World of Electrons

Online abuse—it's almost a dirty term. You are either a victim or a predator, and if you're neither, you are, at the very least, subjected to the extreme negativity it breeds. We have reached a point where people derive pleasure from irking others and by being malicious for no real reason. These electrons, charged with negative energies, are not just ruining their own lives, but are also destroying the peace of everyone around them.

As a celebrity, the moment you decide to make your posts available to the public, you've opened the door to the harsh world of online abuse. There's simply no escaping it. I have personally gone through cycles of dismissal, denial, anger and acceptance in this area. Let me tell you about a few particular incidents to show you things from my perspective.

At the outset, I'd like to say that fans and admirers are like the air that I breathe. I do everything that I do, and continue to be in my line of work, because of the unconditional love and affection that you give. I crave the applause, those cheers and whistles that I am greeted with every time I enter a public gathering. Your genuine love makes everything worth it: every past failure, every lost opportunity and even every painful incident. You are truly the reason I continue to be in the media industry, despite all the unpleasantness I have to deal with.

There is, on the other end of the spectrum, the other kind of people who zap your energy to bits and crush you. I don't understand why they do this to themselves, let alone going about doing it to other people. It isn't sheer sadism or negative criticism that I'm talking about here; they take the whole idea of attacking another person to new heights. I think you'll understand me better with the following anecdotes.

Almost seven years ago, I received an email from an anonymous individual, whom we shall henceforth refer to as 'C' (for 'creep'). This started out as a normal fan mail . . . or at least, that's what I'd thought. He wrote:

'Hi Ramya,
I love you. In all sincerity—will you marry me?'

As flattering as it was, I didn't think much of it initially and simply left it at that. But from then on, C's mails became more frequent, and the messages became more and more perverted by the day. It was clear that he was fantasizing about me. In his head, the guy was having a full-blown relationship with me. Sometimes, the mails would be about his dirty fantasies. At other times, he'd send violent messages threatening me and asking me to mend my ways—apparently, I belonged to him and some of the things I did would upset him. He seemed to be fairly well-read too, judging from the way he wrote his mails.

He was stalking me online and was keeping track of all the shows I was hosting. He was going completely out of control and invading my personal space—he talked about my outfits and his views on them; expressed his disapproval when I wore something fashionable for my shoots; threatened that he would harm me if I stood any closer to the male co-anchors while hosting a show. He was idolizing me as a product he owned and that belonged only to him! I didn't have the option to block him back then on mails; I simply stopped opening his mails and sent them straight to the recycle bin.

I must mention here that cyberstalking is using the Internet to annoy, harass, and threaten a specific individual and is a punishable offence in India. If a woman faces cyberstalking, she can very well file a complaint in any cybercrime unit online, or police station or even file an FIR.

A few months later, my staff forwarded an email from C informing me that his mother had been admitted to the hospital for a surgery—and that I was to blame (yes, that's exactly what he said!). Apparently, all of this had happened because I hated him so intensely and had wished for terrible things to happen to him and his family. He even threatened me by saying that if anything happened to her he wouldn't hesitate to take revenge. It was at this point that I swiftly closed the email account entirely just to get away from this guy who was completely messed up and was making my life a living hell too.

The next incident occurred in 2018. A few years ago, I woke up on Diwali morning to a deluge of WhatsApp messages and missed calls. When I opened the texts, I saw screenshots of tweets that I had no clue about, along with the question: 'Was it you who tweeted this?' Unable to make head or tail of what was going on, I logged on to my Twitter account and got the shock of my life. My account had been hacked, and there was a tweet about the release of a film that day (within one hour of its release!)—how its box office collections had broken the record of another big hero's previous film, and how the star of this film was the undisputed king of the box office. The grammar was terrible, the words were crass and the sentiment was unpleasant . . . it didn't remotely resemble a tweet I'd have made.

The silver lining here was that nobody in the media circle, including the two big stars who were named, paid any attention to this. They all knew me well enough to realize that I'd fallen prey to online abuse and were gracious enough to handle the issue with tact and sensitivity. Despite my efforts to delete the tweet and file a complaint with the Cyber Crime Cell in Chennai, the damage had already been done. The tweet had been retweeted and shared several thousand times by other electrons, and a war of words had broken out between them. For the fans who had a constant rivalry about who the bigger star of the two was, I became the centre of the battle that day; so on one end, abuses were being hurled at me and on the other, I was being praised for my act!

What did I learn from all of this? To make stronger passwords, of course!

But why did I have to face an act of such hostility in the first place? This is just a small example from my numerous encounters on social media, and this is the sort of threat that we are constantly exposed to.

Instagram is more relaxed, in a way. Since they have a system that prioritizes the comments of those whom you follow, and those who follow you, I tend to look at just the comments that pop up first. The flip side of this is that I sometimes miss out on the genuine love and feedback from those who reach out and offer positivity. So now, my social media team filters and sends me screenshots of the positive comments and messages that they think I should know about, and I make it a point to reply to them whenever I can.

Most predators create a fake profile with fake details. The anonymity becomes a shield that enables them to say whatever they like, without any filter or fear of counter-attack, and without shame or dignity. Blocking them is not a pragmatic solution when your following is large, and the more you do it, the more vulnerable you make yourself to the community of electrons. I don't like getting back at the predators either. It's a way of giving them unnecessary attention, and is a waste of my precious time and energy that could be spent on something else. Be aware that this is a criminal offence and if anyone has experienced anything similar from an online predator, you have every right to make a complaint online or in person at the Cyber Crime Cell closest to you and get them put behind bars.

I'm certainly open to constructive criticism. As a public personality in the entertainment industry, I'm bound to get feedback on my work, and that's only fair. The problem is when these boundaries are crossed and the comments go beyond our work, when criticism turns into abuse through harsh words, abusive language and sexual innuendos, as a way of maligning people, seeking attention or gaining some kind of sadistic pleasure.

On certain Instagram posts or YouTube videos about encouraging people to eat healthy and train hard, there have been multiple times where my message has been diluted and brought down to petty topics, and people have left comments to just attack me and pull me down.

For instance, if I say that you should be mindful of fruits and have them in the right proportions as they can spike your blood sugar levels, there will be someone questioning why and how I could promote the idea that eating fruits was bad. If I say that macro counting has given me a lot of insight about nutrition and helps me balance my eating every day, there will be someone saying that 'it leads to toxic eating disorder and obsessing over food portions is not good'. This might be true, and I would respect that and respond by saying that this method may not be for them, leaving them to pursue something else—but if something works for me, why would you spend your time convincing me and my audience to not try it? I have nowhere in this book or even outside in any of my own wellness programs on Stay Fit With Ramya endorsed a specific approach to eating and workouts. I thoroughly believe in the concept of bio individuality when it comes to any aspect of wellness—diet, training, skin, hair regime and more. I do not enforce or endorse an unhealthy/obsessive relationship with food. Macro counting has worked for me in my experience. At the same time, I don't apply this to every client in my own coaching space. I understand where they come from and their past eating habits before coming up with a strategy that works for them. It is funny sometimes thinking even how the smallest of things tend to get misconstrued. 'Lifting weights won't make you big, but your cupcakes may', is a fun quirky caption for 99.9 per cent of the population. The intention in the line is to encourage women who fear weight training to go train and to worry less about 'looking big', but you might not know that there exists a 0.01 per cent who will twist my message and ask how I could spread the idea that we should not eat cupcakes. I used to be baffled and now I find it fascinating how their mind can find fault even in the best of things.

I am not just talking about social media followers here. I know people who share the Instagram posts of someone they follow with their friends on common WhatsApp groups. Dissecting and sabotaging those posts are daily practices that they enjoy. I found it extremely hard to coexist with this crowd and then started making my circle smaller and smaller. I have observed that this urge to put another person down comes from a place of jealousy and frustration. Why not unfriend and unfollow the person whose thoughts you don't agree with and leave it there? Or if you are a friend, why not message the person and tell them what you think in a nice way and make them understand your perspective if you have the right intentions?

The person on the other side of the screen is human too and has feelings, just like you do. So, if you have vented at and judged someone in the past, all I am asking you to do is to think carefully about this course of action the next time you have the urge to put up an angry post, meme, comment or even share their post and make a mockery of it in a private WhatsApp group.

Exercise

Think of someone in your life whose company you don't enjoy, but whom you don't have a choice of staying away from either. It can be a family member, a friend, a colleague or even your boss. Write down three things you like about them below:

1. _____
2. _____
3. _____

Now, the next time you meet them, focus on these qualities instead.

41

When My Life
Became a Rajinikanth Film

While we wake up each day believing that the day ahead is going to be great and feel the courage, strength, compassion and love in us to conquer it and make it our own, not every single day works in our favour. We have good days, bad days and mediocre days. That is how life is sometimes—and that's okay. Since the pandemic especially, I have noticed the increasing importance of mental health, and a lot of men and women keep writing to me about their suffering. More often than not, these issues trail back to a person who had hurt them and overcoming them has been very challenging. While I can't put myself into anyone else's shoes, I can only share how I turned my hurt and my rejections into a response that helped protect my emotional health. Here are two anecdotes. I hope they help you think about better ways of handling your pain.

2013: Chennai

This was when I was in the prime of my hosting days. I was the go-to person for every film producer to host their audio launch, every television producer to host their programme and every event company to emcee their corporate events. I was in a very happy space—working in full swing, doing my best at what I love most—I couldn't possibly have asked for anything better.

But what you see from the outside is never exactly reflective of what is happening within. As you rise up the ladder, the number of people who envy you rises too, sadly. Most of the time, it might not even be obvious to you—people are skilled at acting like they're your best friends to your face, all the while pulling you down behind your back.

There is one such incident I recall from the year 2013. I had been hosting the curtain-raiser for a popular award show for a couple of years continuously before that, so I'd assumed I'd be handling the proceedings for that year too. I even cancelled a few other commitments for other events that coincided with this particular one, just to make room for it in my calendar. I waited and waited for the organizers to call and confirm that I would be hosting it. We were getting closer to the actual date of the event, and the complete silence was starting to get to me.

Meanwhile, my friends and family, who also assumed that I'd be hosting the event just like in the previous years, began asking me for complimentary passes. But there I was, too embarrassed to tell them that I hadn't even received a word about the event! The day of the event came and went by, and

I still had absolutely no clue as to why I had been cut out that year without any information or intimation.

About a month later, I heard a 'scoop' from one of my friends and a colleague who was working in the same firm—a certain someone who wasn't particularly fond of me and had some influence over the decision-making process had strongly opposed my participation that year for no valid reason. This person had done everything in their power to ensure that I was replaced by someone else. To this day, I still don't know why they had a problem with me. I'd met them a number of times before, and even after this episode, we've exchanged pleasantries and our encounters have always been friendly. While at times I used to think if I should confront them and check on what their exact issue with me was and see if I can amicably settle it out, even if I were to confront them, what could I possibly say? I certainly couldn't reveal the name of the one person who had trusted me and shared this information with me.

This incident was a wake-up call for me to realize that there are mostly no real friends in the world of media. I take my time with growing attached to people after this incident, and don't open up too easily with everyone. My self-love has become much stronger than my desire for work or the desire to be loved by others, and the truth I realized is that not everyone will love us in the real world anyway.

With all the sudden twists and changing decisions on everything that keeps happening like a rollercoaster in the media world at the spur of a moment, I have now finally settled myself with the most profound understanding that no one can take what is meant for me, and I don't want what was meant for someone else. So, no excitement or disappointment in my world today over anything. It is what it is.

2014: Geneva, Switzerland

I was to host a huge event in Geneva and had checked into the accommodation provided to me by the show organizer.

It was a tiny single room, so tiny that there wasn't even enough space for my luggage. I had to dump all of it right in front of the main door and that completely blocked my way. I also had to bend each time I entered the tinier bathroom, or else I'd bang my head on the ceiling! It was such a claustrophobic experience. I drew the curtains to get a glimpse of the view outside—it was dark and gloomy, and even though it was only 4 p.m., there wasn't a single car or person on the road. I had a sinking feeling in my stomach and tears pricked my eyes. I felt lonely, missed my family, and I hadn't even eaten a proper meal in about 15 hours. There I was, in this ridiculously tiny room where I couldn't even freshen up. I tripped over my luggage and fell onto the single bed. I don't remember anything after that.

A few hours later, I heard the doorbell ring. It was the organizer. He greeted me warmly, but I bet he noticed my eyes, which were completely red and swollen by then. He quickly apologized about the room, assuring me that there had been a mix-up. He told me that we were leaving immediately, and then he put me up at another hotel. Anything I saw after that experience was divine in comparison. Seeing the faces of my other colleagues who had travelled from India for the same show lifted my spirits too. The event was successful, and

I received a lot of appreciation from everyone at the end of the evening.

The same organizer came up to me elated afterwards and thanked me for hosting the event successfully. He then hesitated before confessing to me that he had wanted to book the larger hotel room for me to begin with, but that a certain film producer (who had been part of the event) had felt that I was being given too much importance. A mere anchor didn't deserve to be put up in the same hotel as the rest of them. I hadn't reached their level apparently, and so I deserved a smaller place. I smiled, keeping all the hurt inside me, and just thanked him for believing in me and reserving a better place for me while we were in a new country.

In 2018, I went to one of the BMW showrooms in Chennai to buy a car, using all my hard-earned savings from the last few years. This was a special moment that I wanted to celebrate with my parents, so they came along too. Guess whom we bumped into? The same producer who had said that I didn't deserve to be on par with him!

I was sitting in the driver's seat in one of the cars. A sales representative was tutoring me on the controls of the car for a test drive, when the producer peeped in through the window. He was shocked to see me. I stepped out of the car, said hi to him and asked him what he was doing there. He had come to buy a car for his daughter who was going to college, and rather liked the colour of the car I was in. I told him that I was there to gift a car to my parents with the money I had earned through a lot of hard work.

There was a moment of silence. The expression on his face quickly changed, and that was my winning moment. I could tell that he felt guilty about what he had said all those years ago, and for judging me based on some unwritten rules of hierarchy. I thanked the gods for making our paths cross again at that exact time. Money and fame say nothing about a person's worth, and no one should judge or put anyone in hierarchy based on them. That was not just his lesson, but mine too.

The Geneva incident didn't bother me for more than a few days, and I had absolutely no plans to go buy the exact same car that he had wanted on that same date and time years afterwards just to teach him a lesson, but our paths just crossed with perfect timing. I felt the hurt I had gone through back then had manifested this way for him to sense his wrongdoing.

Have you realized that people look very different when we don't care for them or respect them anymore? We realize how ordinary they are, and how it was due to our impressions that we had placed them on a pedestal. We need to observe people with that attitude, more closely, and sooner rather than later decide whom we want as part of our story, and who all are meant to be reduced to only a chapter!

Also, while talking about people and their impact on our mental health, I have always felt that while you and I are not responsible for something bad that happens to us, we are responsible for breaking that cycle and not hurting more people around us just because of what happened to us. I have seen the difference: I am a much nicer person to those around me when I am happier. This means that holding onto what or who hurt us is not going to help us be a better person for our own self and well-being. This also says a lot about the people who aren't very nice to us. I wish them well while getting on my way.

If you are in pain because of some work or personal relationship right now, I pray that whatever is hurting you gets better, and that you overcome all overthinking and dark thoughts with clarity, calmness, love and peace.

Exercise

Remember a time when a certain situation unfolded beautifully in your favour, all on its own. I'm going to spare you from writing about it. Just remember it and relive your 'superstar' moment.

_____

_____

_____

Epilogue

Last but Not the Least

Thus, we have come to the end of the book . . . I hope you've enjoyed reading it!

Firstly, thank you for giving me your time and the opportunity to share my experiences. I am grateful and truly humbled for in this crazy busy time of life when technology has completely taken over our lives, reading a book takes a lot of effort and patience, and you did that trusting in me and my first-time writing experience as an author.

I shared a lot of my own stories in this book, some for the very first time, simply because I wanted you to get to know 'Ramya the person', beyond 'Ramya the Media Personality or Fitness Enthusiast'.

As you now know, things haven't always been rosy for me. I've had to fight several battles, repeatedly pull myself together and get things done. I've had my share of dark days, but they always turned around whenever I decided to focus on making it a better day. I believe that we as humans are made to push boundaries, break that tight cork open and get out of our comfort zone. Only if we make that effort can we see life change before us in the ways that we want it to—so go ahead and do it! This is what I've learnt from my personal experiences.

Whenever I have faced complicated situations, I think of it like a video game level from the outside, and find ways to get out of them rather than be trapped inside and suffocate. We do have the strength and ability to swim through the challenges and come out in one piece.

When we show life that we are capable, won't give up easily, and that we truly deserve to be happy, it will reciprocate, just give it that time . . . Life has always done it for me. Then I look back, smile and say 'yes, I got that done!'

If I could do it, so can you.

I want you to accomplish all the goals you've set for yourself, be it fitness or life goals. I genuinely believe that you can achieve them. Yes, there would be some hit and miss situations, our inner spirits may knock us down and we tend to get discouraged but amidst all that, you are the most powerful person in your life and it should always be you calling the shots. And I hope that in some small way, this book will serve as inspiration for you to keep remembering that. The ride won't be easy and it's important to enjoy the journey to ensure that the the end destination is worth it. I would love to hear your thoughts on this book for it would encourage me to do more and learn more in my own life going forward. You know where to reach me; hit me up on my social media accounts which I have mentioned below. It would be lovely to see more of you with me there too. So, if you haven't been following me there already, please do so now and I'll catch up with you.

If you are interested in my fitness programmes (ladies only) that I currently run online, start following me on Instagram: @stayfitwithramya

Check out my website: https://stayfitwithramya.exlyapp.com/.

Sweat it out, become disciplined, give yourself constant reality checks and just keep making heads turn. We have one life and I'm rooting for you with all my heart to have a magical one.

With love,

Ramya

youtube.com/c/StayfitwithRamya
Instagram: @ramyasub @stayfitwithramya
Twitter: @actorramya
Facebook.com/VJRamyaOfficial

Acknowledgements

No one achieves anything alone. According to me, every person who steps foot in your path, even just a tiny toe, serves a purpose in your life. I have had the pleasure of meeting hundreds of people as a result of my wide exposure in the media world and outside, and each of them have influenced the thoughts that I hold deep and strong in my life. The heartfelt conversations I have had with the people who have deeply impacted me, all of the hugs, the laughs, the smiles and the tears we have shared and the learnings I have experienced in this time have shaped me into who I am today.

To the One above me, without Whom I couldn't have had this life that I'm hustling my way through, thank You for blessing me with the best of everything in abundance and always treating me as one of Your favourite creations. I am what I am only because of Your creation. I almost feel like Your favourite child from the way You let me face obstacles in my journey but dive in at the right time to take control to protect me. I believe Your timing has always been right in everything that has happened to me and this is why I continue to have blind faith always in You.

In a way, writing this book was like pressing a reset button after living through the majority of the years until now without taking a pause, reflecting on the beautiful and not-so-beautiful moments before carrying forward with the lessons I learnt. I have been in a bubble and it was the couple of years during the COVID-19 lockdown with little or no contact with anyone else when things hit me hard and I realized I had to value the people in my life more. There is no appropriate word to describe how perfect the timing to write this book was.

Thank you!

My superpowers in human forms, Amma and Appa. Just thinking about you makes me emotional. You have both prioritized and continue to choose me over anything and everything else. Thank you for the countless sacrifices for me, for your understanding, for keeping me grounded and for bringing me up with the right kind of values and discipline. Thank you for letting your crazy daughter follow her crazy dreams and for having the guts to give me the freedom to do what I believed in amidst all adversity.

Most importantly, I love you and you mean the entire world and the universe and the Heaven (hopefully if I end up there) and all the rest put together to me.

Thank you to my brother Deepak, for being the silent and hardworking one. Thank you for raising the bar for me to keeping pushing to perform better and excel, to keep up with you. I will always look up to you.

KV, I know you don't like it when I say 'thank you' to you, but pardon me this time, considering I am not doing it to your face right now. Friends like you don't just happen to everyone. From being my nearest and dearest, to being a rock and holding on to me during the rollercoaster rides I face day in and out, you support me in ways I can never understand. It was you who suggested I write my life experiences in the form of a book when I was sulking to you one day about my boredom during the lockdown. Can you believe this has happened now, and today if I may call myself an author (all authors around kindly excuse me on this), it is ONLY because of YOU!

To my friend and nurturer, director Raj Kumar Periasamy. While in the media world, men may come and men may go, you are that one solid, sorted friend who I know will stay on forever. Thank you for being just a call away always and helping me handle the toughest transitions with both your intellect and humour.

Abi Senguttuvan, my head nutritionist and dear friend now, you entered my life with a random Instagram DM and little did I know then that you will occupy such a big role in working along with me on Stay Fit With Ramya. You know how hard it is behind the scenes for me being an entrepreneur, student, actor, anchor, social media influencer and author. Every time I broke down, overwhelmed with work and anxiety, you have lifted me up so selflessly. You are a true 'always and forever' person sent to me by God. To us always being Happily Fit!

Sandya and Sriram, I call you mommy and daddy not just for the fun part but also because I know you are there for me and care of me and think of my happiness so much. DC, my gym partner, on-the-go photographer and gadget guru, you have transformed the girl who didn't know how to load a SIM card into her phone into someone who can pay all her utility bills online on her own without guidance today. How cool are you.

Thank you to my coach and friend Jyotsna. I honestly think that I wouldn't have developed this passion for fitness if I hadn't met you at the right time. You patiently guided me in the same career as you, despite being in such a competitive space like the fitness industry. It goes to show how secure and generous you are as a coach and as a person.

Sadhana, I still remember seeing you from the stage pray for me real hard with your eyes closed tightly to see me win the title in the Miss Chennai Beauty Pageant, while sitting next to my mom. I know you feel like you win when you see me win. Chithu, I haven't forgotten you. You are a warrior and you inspire me with the way you smile in between everything that life throws at you. Love you both.

To every other friend too who I can't name in this limited space, I just want to say that you have helped me become a better person with every passing day. I truly cherish our friendship and wish you nothing but the best.

Thank you, dear Aruna Vijay, culinary enthusiast, for instantly agreeing when I asked if you would prepare the recipes for this book and for wholeheartedly working on it, meticulously curating some wonderful recipes for our book. Your love for cooking amazes me. So glad you are part of this one.

A lot of women who have been a part of my life in different ways have been responsible for instilling in me a hustler mindset, without them even knowing it. This included even the clients I coach day in and out. I admire each of you for how great you are in own your lives irrespective of whatever challenges come in the way. I need to mention this here for you are helping me get to where I am today and will grow to be tomorrow, just by setting an example with the way you lead your life.

Thank you, my biggest inspirations (in no order of preference):

Sam (actor Samantha) for being a hustler and taking me along with you. The way you relentlessly chase your goals always inspires me. You being exactly the same as you always are despite anything and everything is the best part about you.

Dr Priya Selvaraj (fertility specialist) for being the incredible mom, doctor, friend, excellent cook, fabulous yogini and always finding the time to learn more and do more! You mean so much to me and I know that you know it too.

Dr Renita Rajan (dermatologist), I have been drawn to your kindness, charm and personality from the day I met you, like a magnet. The glow that shines from within you is what reflects on us, your patients. Keep shining.

Hasini Ma'am (Mrs Suhasini Maniratnam) for being a unicorn, always accomplishing and being so effortlessly talented, so multifaceted, making me feel the value of the milliseconds in every second.

Trashers (actor Trisha), I remember you telling me during the lockdown that you wished I was conducting personal sessions and coaching clients for you to have enrolled, and you set my mind rolling that day. Whatever I planned and did since then to become a health coach today was keeping in mind the words you encouraged me with.

You are a gem. So simple and grounded no matter how much you achieve.

I'm almost done, don't worry.

Thank you, Praveena. You were the first one to read the notes I scribbled down and to tell me that it was a workable manuscript that could potentially become a published book. As a writer yourself, it was your initial positive words that gave me the confidence to turn these jottings into a book. I owe it to you for introducing me to Poonam Ganglani, who gave me her perspective on what worked in my manuscript and what could be improved, to turn it into an appealing finished product. Your observations worked big time Poonam. Thank you.

Thank you, team Penguin Random House India for instantly responding to the proposal mail I sent you by immediately saying YES! It gives me goosebumps even today and I have starred that first mail I received from you. Being a huge lover of the books released by PRH, I had manifested for this to happen and I am forever grateful to you for making me an author. To more books in the future!

My editors at Penguin, Shreya Punj and Rea Mukherjee, thank you for having my back throughout this entire book-writing process, guiding me stage by stage, encouraging my work and being so supportive of everything to make my dream become a reality today.

Thank you to each of my other trainers and dietician friends for sharing your knowledge and experiences, and for helping me gain insights into the subject of wellness.

A big thank you to all my friends in the media and, most importantly, my fans who have showered me with love and kind words for the last few years, especially in the area of fitness. The way you responded to my transformation gave me all the courage and confidence to make this my career too, and a part of that is this book. Thank you for always jumping in and signing up for my coaching programmes, workshops and everything to which I started out believing that I would add the value you sought. Thank you for accepting me and giving me a place in your heart. More than love, it is the respect that I feel you have for me that makes me want to grow stronger and live up to it. No matter what I would have or not tomorrow, the one thing I know I can fall back on at anytime in this lifetime is your unconditional love and cheers for me always. I am grateful to you all eternally for you are the wind beneath my wings and what I am today is only because you chose me from among so many others who wanted to be in my place.

Now I know exactly why the acceptance speeches in award functions sound so long to others but not to the one doing the talking . . . because one can't skip nor miss any important names, and most of all because it can get frigging long!